PENGUIN BOOKS
Annie's Coming Out

Rosemary Crossley was born in a country town in Victoria, Australia, in 1945 and received her B.A. at the National University in Canberra in 1966. She worked in the commonwealth public service as a research assistant and computer programmer before leaving to go overseas in 1970. On her return in 1971 she worked for two years at the Dame Mary Herring Spastic Centre in Melbourne. In 1974 she took up a position at St Nicholas Hospital in Melbourne and worked there for the next five years, during which she took a Diploma of Education. In 1980 she was transferred to the Health Commission Library. In 1982 she resigned to work at home with Anne McDonald. Since early 1984 she has been a teacher with the Spastic Society.

Anne McDonald was born in a small town, also in the country in Victoria, in 1961. Disabled by cerebral palsy at birth, she was placed in St Nicholas Hospital in Melbourne at the age of three. She remained there until her eighteenth birthday, when she left and went to live in Rosemary Crossley's home in Melbourne. She has currently interrupted a university course to work on a book about ethics and disability with the assistance of a grant from the Australia Council.

ANNIE'S COMING OUT
Rosemary Crossley
and Anne McDonald

PENGUIN BOOKS

Penguin Books Ltd, Harmondsworth, Middlesex, England
Viking Penguin Inc., 40 West 23rd Street, New York, New York 10010, U.S.A.
Penguin Books Australia Ltd, Ringwood, Victoria, Australia
Penguin Books Canada Ltd, 2801 John Street, Markham, Ontario, Canada L3R 1B4
Penguin Books (N.Z.) Ltd, 182–190 Wairau Road, Auckland 10, New Zealand

First published by Penguin Books Australia 1980
Published in Pelican Books in Great Britain 1982
Reprinted with revisions in Penguin Books 1984

Copyright © Rosemary Crossley and Anne McDonald, 1980, 1984
All rights reserved

Printed and bound in Great Britain by
Cox & Wyman Ltd, Reading
Set in Century Old Style

Photographs of Anne McDonald and Rosemary Crossley (p. vi)
reprinted with permission of the *Age*, Melbourne. Photograph of Anne
McDonald (p. 253) by Alex Bauer.

Except in the United States of America, this book is sold subject
to the condition that it shall not, by way of trade or otherwise, be lent,
re-sold, hired out, or otherwise circulated without the
publisher's prior consent in any form of binding or cover other than
that in which it is published and without a similar condition
including this condition being imposed on the subsequent purchaser

TO:

MARK ANDERSON
LEONIE MCFARLANE
PHILLIP MARMO
NOELENE MORGAN
SHARON PERTZEL
ANGELA PUGLIELLI
SHIRLEY STEELE
ANGELA WALLACE

and to

MARK CORKHILL
STEPHEN CUNLIFFE
DENNIS MORRIS
LESLEY WADDINGHAM

who did not live to come out

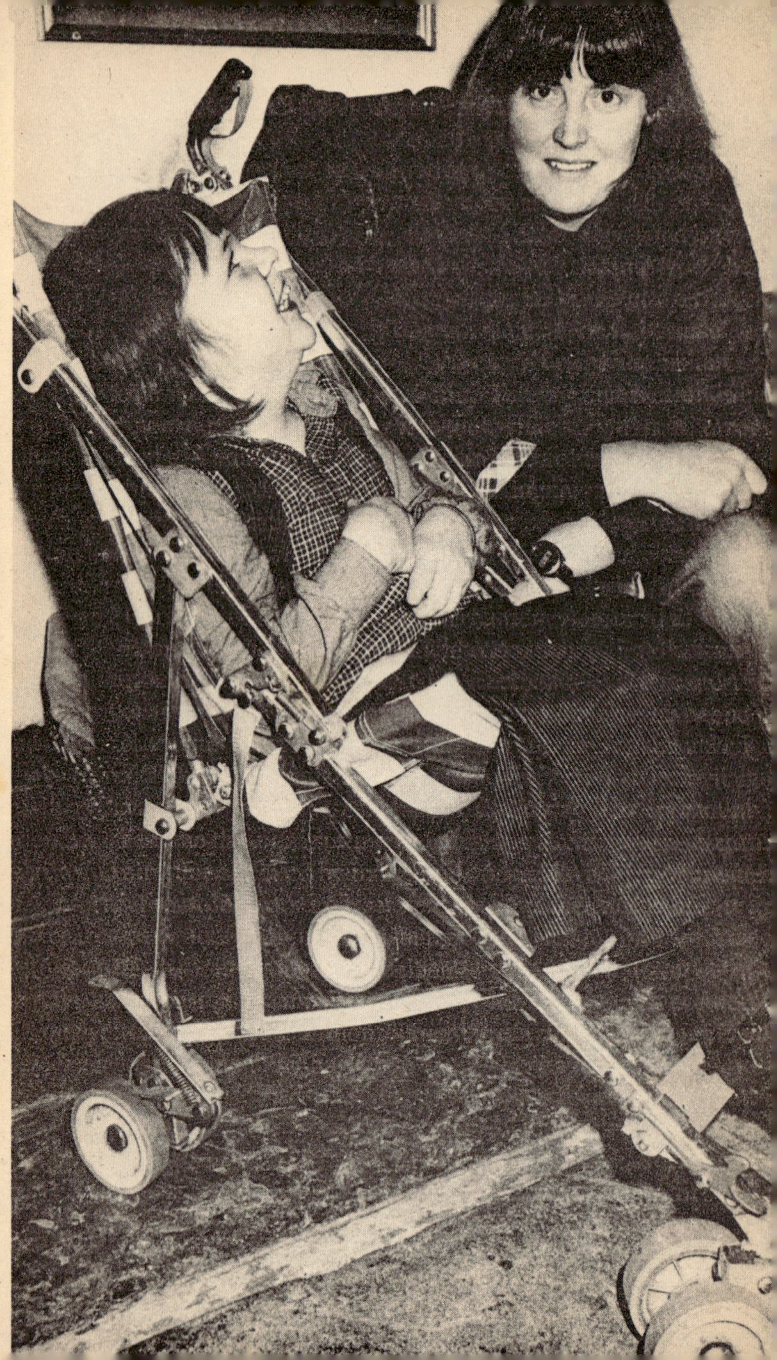

To be imprisoned inside one's own body is dreadful. To be confined in an institution for the profoundly retarded does not crush you in the same way; it just removes all hope.

I went to St Nicholas Hospital when I was three. The hospital was the state garbage bin. Very young children were taken into permanent care, regardless of their intelligence. If they were disfigured, distorted, or disturbed then the world should not have to see or acknowledge them. You knew that you had failed to measure up to the standard expected of babies. You were expected to die.

Never seeing normal children, we were not sure what they were like. Where did we fall short? In your ugly body it was totally impossible that there could be a mind. Vital signs showed that your title was 'human'; but that did not entitle you to live like normal children. You were totally outside the boundary which delineated the human race.   ANNE McDONALD

Foreword

Heroine or humbug? Saviour of repressed institutionalized children or fanatical agitator in a fine and caring hospital for crippled and retarded young persons? These are the extreme views that Rosemary Crossley aroused in Melbourne's St Nicholas Hospital, the Health Commission of Victoria, and in the Australian community at large over her long fight to have her protégée Anne McDonald declared to be no longer an infirm person and, having reached maturity at the age of eighteen, free to make her own decisions about her lifestyle and her right to leave St Nicholas.

A foreword to a book is not the place to make judgements about its authors. Anyhow this has already been done. The Supreme Court, before the Honourable Mr Justice Jenkinson on 19 May 1979, and before the Honourable Justice Murphy on 25 September 1979, found Anne McDonald to be competent to manage her own affairs, thus absolving Rosemary Crossley of the charge that she manipulated Annie's arm to spell out answers to questions from an alphabet board. A Committee of Enquiry set up by the Health Commission to examine Ms Crossley's allegation that at least eleven other severely handicapped children at St Nicholas were also intelligent found this to be not so and that Rosemary's activities were so divisive of staff and disruptive of patient care at St Nicholas that she should no longer work there. On this advice the Health Commission transferred Rosemary Crossley from St Nicholas, so severing her contact with her other protégés.

In spite of the bitterness surrounding it, Rosemary's story of her long, patient battle to establish communication with Anne is human and moving. That process of unlocking a real human being, with senses, feelings and thoughts, is a magnificent accomplishment of patience, perseverence, and innovation.

Restraints and lack of stimulation are often characteristic of institutions. In the conflict between these problems, traditional mental health techniques of assessing an individual's competence and Rosemary's fierce battle to develop the individuality of her charges, the real issue has been lost. That is that medical science has not yet solved the problem of how much severe disorders of communication may mask the observer's ability to detect a real person, a unique individual behind the wall of gross deformity, uncontrollable movement and noises that do not resemble speech. Unhappily, medical science shows little evidence of coming to grips with the issue, preferring to develop human dumping grounds, calling them long-term wards or convalescent units. Further, there is my own profession's tendency to label human beings, for example, as 'dements', 'vegetables', 'retarded', 'schizophrenic'. Such terms tend to class the worth of a human being and discourage efforts to discover what even severely brain-damaged people can enjoy: emotions, tastes, sensations and the warmth of a relationship with other people.

Institution is becoming a dirty word in modern society, being associated with gloomy buildings, inferior accommodation, poor facilities, and staff more concerned with the custody of their charges than with their happiness. The stereotype of the institution is one in which the wishes of the residents are not consulted, and their lifestyle is controlled by time-tables and procedures suited to the convenience of the staff, not the inmates. Not all modern institutions are like that, however, and over the last two decades there have been steady reforms in procedures and efforts to make inmates become residents who participate in decisions about what happens to their own lives and bodies. The Mental Health Authority can be well proud of its efforts in this direction, but reforms cannot be made overnight, and there are too many black pockets of decaying institutions in our society, staffed by persons who are given salaries, conditions and status that encourage few reformers of the zeal of Rosemary Crossley to join their ranks.

While reforms on the professional side of institutions go on, society itself has to come to grips with a fundamental reform: that handicapped people are citizens, not patients, and have rights they can demand as well as rules they should obey. The United Nations Declaration of Human Rights enshrines this principle; our government has accepted it. The problem is putting principle into practice.

Reformers, however, come and go. The more outspoken, the more uncompromising, the more troublesome to the authorities they are, those who attack with zeal often kick the system along more rapidly for a while than can the quiet army of patient reformers of nurses and therapists working at the grass-roots, sometimes under local managers and matrons whose attitudes reflect more the management of the Poor House of Victorian times than the modern ideal. The fierce reformers have had their successes, but in the long run the system turns against them and throws them out. So goes Rosemary Crossley.

As any student of sociology knows, social change by its very nature moves slowly, as the process of debate and education of individuals and groups move to a new consensus. The zealot is a necessary ingredient of this process of change: hurrying it along, getting it through bogs, fighting the greatest enemy of all – apathy.

BRUCE FORD, July 1980
Director of Rehabilitation Services, Alfred/Caulfield Hospital, Melbourne

Acknowledgements

Our thanks go especially to Christian Borthwick, without whom this story would not have occurred and without whose help this book would not have been published.

We also wish to thank the Allums; the Assembly and those associated with it; the members of the Beanbaggers Support Group and DEAL; Brian Johns, Jackie Yowell, Geoff Cook, and Kevin Childs; Graham Dethridge, Jon Hamer, Peter Heerey, David Harper, and Chris Grieg; Donna Anderson, Debbie Jones, Kathy Latham, and Lyn Farley-Smith; Kaye Gooch; Philip Graves; John Hickman; Sonia Humphries; the Joneses; Janet McColl; Jean Melzer; the Moores; Katy and Gabrielle Wall and Christobel and Sasha Munson; Jim Patrick; Joy Peletier; Sean O'Connor and Janet Taylor; David Brownridge; Chris Biddle; Mr Puttar; those members of Mental Retardation Services who have given support but who cannot, for their own safety, be thanked by name; the Supreme Court of Victoria; the volunteers and sessional staff who worked with Rosemary at St Nicholas; and all the other people – relatives, friends, politicians and members of the public – who gave us support and sympathy.

Finally we thank our editor, Jane Arms, without whom this book would have been twice as long and half as good.

1980

Preface to Revised Edition

Looking back over *Annie's Coming Out* we can see a lot of things that we would like to change: places where the language is unsuitable (calling the group 'the beanbaggers', for example) or long explanations of communication methods that in the light of what we have learnt since seem rather crude and clumsy. That was how we thought in 1980, however, and the only revision we have made is to rewrite the epilogue to bring the book up to date.

There is one misunderstanding we would like to clear up. In 1980, in an ill-advised attempt to reassure parents who might be concerned about their children who had been at St Nicholas, we said, truthfully, 'Many of the genuinely profoundly retarded children have been happy there.' The sentence was badly phrased and was taken by some people to mean that we thought that conditions at St Nicholas were appropriate for people with profound retardation. This is certainly not the case. Conditions in St Nicholas were not appropriate for anyone.

We would like to thank all the people and organizations who have helped us or the people at St Nicholas since 1980, especially Mary McMenamin, Jude McHenry, Fiona Stewart and Richard Davey and the Salamanca Theatre Company who wrote and produced a play based on *Annie's Coming Out* in Tasmania; Ron Hoenig, Tina Anderssen and the team from Troupe who presented Ron's play based on

Annie's Coming Out in Adelaide; Gil Brealey, Don Murray and all the people at Film Australia; Tina Arhondis and the other players in the film; all the people who supported us and the group at St Nicholas after *Annie's Coming Out* was published; George Winston and the helpers from T.A.D., particularly John Scholten; Bill Hosemans; Mark Snedden, Tim Woods, John Dwyer and all at Mallesons; Errol Cocks and those other M.R.D. staff who have been trying to struggle against the rigidities of the system; Jenny Townsend and other staff at Deakin University; the Principal and staff of University High Evening School; V.I.S.E., V.C.O.S.S., and the D.R.C.; The Australia Council; Dr Robert Cummins, Ms Heather Bancroft, and other staff at Burwood State College; Margaret Batt and Rosemary Ryall; Rhonda Galbally; The Spastic Society; and the Queen Victoria Medical Centre.

Chapter One

Anne was born on 11 January 1961 in a small country town in Victoria, Australia. Her father runs a small business in the town, and her family still lives there. Annie was the second of five children. Her parents are ordinary, intelligent people, and her handicaps are the result of a difficult birth. The pregnancy was unalarming, but she was a breech delivery, which means she came out backside first, and she did not breathe spontaneously after delivery. Within twenty-four hours she was transferred to the Royal Children's Hospital in the state capital, Melbourne. Her medical records say, 'On the second day 4 ml of blood were aspirated from the (L) subdural space and subsequently further amounts were aspirated from both sides. She had intermittent cyanotic attacks, head retraction, and required gavage feeding.' Basically that means that because of an intra-cranial haemorrhage, her early days were stormy.

The difficulties surrounding her birth had left her affected with the athetoid form of cerebral palsy. This means that she had suffered an injury to the brain stem, which is at the base of the brain directly joining the spinal cord. All messages from the brain to the muscles must pass through this area.

If you think of the brain as a large mail order department store, Annie's brain runs like *Sears Roebuck* with a maniac in charge of the despatch department. Incoming messages are received from eyes and ears and processed appropriately. They go to their respective departments and all the operations needed are carried out perfectly. The correct packages with the correct addresses and postage instructions are sent to the despatch department. There everything goes berserk: addresses are wilfully muddled; packages are sent to people who have not asked for them and not sent to people who have. Annie's limbs receive unasked-for messages in turn, resulting in twitching that moves its way around the body, giving her the classic athetoid writhing movement. Her tongue receives unwanted messages which make it push in and out: tongue-thrust is one of the most characteristic manifestations of brain-stem injury. This makes eating and talking very difficult.

These involuntary patterns of movement are with Annie for every waking minute. When she tries to do something herself, the messages get scrambled again. If she tries to move an arm, her head will go back or to one side. If she tries to move her leg and arm, her other leg will probably start to move as well. Every movement involves an enormous uncertainty; even if she does get the right part to move, she cannot be sure how fast or how far it will move, and what is meant to be a small movement can end up dashing crockery off the table in all directions.

When Annie was born her mother was told that her daughter would never be able to do anything. When Annie was discharged from the Royal Children's Hospital she went back with her parents to the country and lived with them and her older brother Ewan for the next three years.

During this time Annie came down to the Royal Children's Hospital from time to time for outpatient appointments with various specialists. On one of these visits she was given the only psychological assessment recorded for the first sixteen years of her life. The report read, in part:

At present, she is showing little progress in development. At the age of 1 year 10 months, she is unable to sit by herself. She requires all the care of a six-months-old baby, though she is showing more alertness and response in her expression and is able to grasp objects for short periods.

The writer did not suggest that Anne was intellectually retarded.

It is always difficult to assess the intellectual capacity of very young children. The standard 'psychological' tests for babies and toddlers are performance tests: the child is assessed on what skills he has, and when he achieves them; on whether he can sit unsupported, or walk, or perform certain tasks such as stacking blocks on the instructions of the psychologist. Such tests obviously cannot be used to assess the intellectual abilities of a child who is too physically handicapped to be able to do them. The psychologist who wrote the report showed herself to be aware of these difficulties and did not write Annie off as retarded simply because of the problems of assessing her with standard measures.

St Nicholas Hospital was officially opened on 13 December 1964 but received its first patients several days earlier. Annie was one of them. The referral to St Nicholas had been suggested by an orthopaedic surgeon at the Royal Children's Hospital. A letter of referral from her family's general practitioner described her as 'a retarded, spastic child'. There is no record of her having been seen by any doctor or psychologist from the Mental Health Authority, the state government body responsible for the provision of services for the psychiatrically ill and the mentally retarded, before she was presented for admission.

In putting Annie into St Nicholas her parents were acting on the best medical advice open to them, and they cannot be criticized for taking that step. Even now, Victoria offers very little in the way of help for handicapped children living at home. In 1964 there was almost no formal help available, and the responsibility for full, twenty-four-hour care for a dependent child rested entirely on the parents. The concept of large institutions had not yet been discredited, and St Nicholas was to be a show-place. It was to provide the therapy, modern equipment, and high-powered medical treatment which was lacking in the country. Annie's parents could not have known that St Nicholas Hospital would not honour its promises.

St Nicholas is housed in the former buildings of the Children's Hospital. When the Children's Hospital moved into new buildings in Royal Park it bequeathed the old ones to the Mental Health Authority. The Mental Health Authority refurbished some of the old buildings, demolished others, and announced the opening of a short-stay residential hospital for very young severely and profoundly retarded children with physical handicaps. By definition profoundly retarded people have IQs of less than 20; severely retarded people have IQs ranging between 20 and 35.

Originally St Nicholas was conceived as a hospital where children could come for a few weeks to give their parents a break from the pressure of full-time care, and the age limit was set at eight. There was an acute shortage of residential accommodation in Victoria for the handicapped, however, and the idea of temporary stays soon went largely by the board. Most of St Nicholas's residents came there and did not go home.

The four wards housing the children were in two substantial Queen Anne buildings dating from the 1890s: three-storey, red brick buildings with balconies that had been enclosed to provide more space. The hospital, named after the patron saint of children, is in Carlton, an inner-city suburb of Melbourne, and it is surrounded by high brick walls topped with barbed wire and broken glass. Inside the hospital some buildings had been demolished and some small lawns planted, but as St Nicholas was designed to cater for only a small number of children, there was space to build a number of administrative facilities; an assessment centre and a sheltered workshop for retarded adults living at home were added.

St Nicholas was not a hospital suited to intelligent people, but many of the genuinely profoundly retarded children have been happy there, and many of the deprivations which meant so much to Annie affected them only slightly. It was not expected that Annie would live very long; many seriously handicapped children did not. The implications of the antibiotic revolution had not been fully realized.

When Annie came to St Nicholas in 1964 I was in the second year of a Bachelor of Arts degree at the Australian National University in Canberra. I was nineteen. My mother had died at the time of my birth, and my home was with my father and stepmother on a farm in Victoria. I finished my degree at the end of 1966 and applied for a job in the public service. While I was waiting for it I took a holiday job at the Dame Mary Herring Spastic Centre in Melbourne. That was my first real encounter with physically handicapped people.

I found the work fascinating, but at that stage I thought of it as no more than a holiday job. I went back to Canberra to work, and I spent the next few years as a research officer. In 1969 I did a computer programming course, and in 1970 I worked in the programming section of the Commonwealth Department of Health. I kept thinking back to the time I had spent at the Spastic Centre, and reflected how much more I had enjoyed the work I had been doing then than anything I had done since.

Disillusioned with programming, I set off for England to study or work with physically handicapped people. Visa restrictions made this impossible and I returned to Australia after fifteen months. While waiting for a job back at the

Spastic Centre, I was interviewed for a job as a ward assistant at St Nicholas.

I remember the place vividly. The woman who interviewed me had difficulty in accepting that I was really interested in the work and would stay for more than a month. To test my sincerity she took me on a tour of the hospital. If anything would put me off, she thought, that would.

It was an afternoon in the middle of summer, and sunlight was streaming through the windows. In the first ward we went to all the children except two were lying in their cots, which filled the dormitory. The two who were not in bed – two toddlers with Down's syndrome – were all by themselves in an enormous and completely bare playroom. It had a highly polished white vinyl floor, and white vinyl ran up the base of the walls. The windows were so high you could not see out of them, and there was absolutely nothing else; not a toy in sight. It was depressing, but I persisted. I did want to work there, I said. I had been accepted and was to start there in a week's time when I heard that there was a position for me at the Spastic Centre. I took up my job there at the beginning of 1972.

I am glad now that I did not go to St Nicholas in 1972. The experience I got at the Spastic Centre in the next two years was invaluable. I came up against a wide range of physically handicapped people with all degrees of physical and mental handicap. Some of the most physically handicapped people were among the most intelligent, and some of the most physically able were profoundly retarded. I met a number of very seriously handicapped and intelligent athetoids and became familiar with their involuntary movement pattern. I worked in the junior section at the Spastic Centre and was responsible for a small group of children each year: a very intellectually handicapped group in the first year, a more intellectually able group in the second.

My time there was important in shaping my future attitudes. The staff there made it clear that each person with cerebral palsy was an individual. They did not conclude: 'Can't walk, can't talk, can't be intelligent.' The centre's therapy and education had enabled many adults who could neither walk nor talk to show that they were just as intelligent as adults who could do both, sometimes more so. There was a good ratio of therapists to trainees, and a certain amount of therapy was considered the right of every person no matter how mentally or physically handicapped. Every effort was made to help the children to achieve those self-help skills that would make life easier for their parents.

I learnt a great deal from the therapists. They could explain why a spastic automatically pulled against you if you pulled her foot to straighten her leg. And they could suggest other ways of manipulating her that would have the desired effect. In addition to developing movement skills, the physiotherapists were particularly concerned with positioning those children who were so physically handicapped that they were never going to be able to walk or move around unaided. The occupational therapists were concerned with developing hand skills and had cunning ways to enable physically handicapped children to participate in the same kinds of activities as other children. They had ways of adapting paint brushes, for example, to make them easier to hold, or different ways of painting so that you did not have to hold anything. They had ways of adapting games so that everybody, including the children without speech, could join in. The availability of special equipment was taken for granted. Both children and adults were expected to conform as far as possible to ordinary rules of behaviour: staff called the children by their first names, asked them politely to do things, did not talk about them in front of them, and in general treated them as ordinary children except where some allowance had to be made for mental handicap.

My father died towards the end of 1972, and I inherited enough from his estate to be able to think about doing a full-time training course in 1974. I was accepted for a course at the Institute of Early Childhood Development, and I resigned from my job at the Spastic Centre. As it happened, the course I wanted to take was cancelled two weeks before it was due to start, and I was left out on a limb: no job to go back to and no time to apply for another training course.

I had met Jean Vant, the Mental Health Authority's Senior Psychologist, when she had brought students to visit the Spastic Centre, and I knew that she was in charge of training teachers to work in the Day Training Centres, which the Mental Health Authority ran for moderately retarded children. (At that time retarded children fell outside the charter of the Education Department.) I rang her to ask if there had been any last-minute vacancies in her course. There were not any vacancies, but she did offer me a job.

She needed an assistant to help run the course, and she asked me if I could start the next day. I agreed thankfully, and at the end of February 1974 I went to work for Mental Deficiency Training Services. Mental Deficiency Training Services was based at St Nicholas Hospital.

In 1975 I wrote a submission for a Committee of Inquiry the Premier of Victoria had set up into mental retardation services. I was not trying to single out St Nicholas – most of the other Mental Health Authority institutions had similar problems – but my account of life in an institution describes Annie's life at that time fairly well.

Stone walls do not a prison make, nor iron bars a cage; they do, however, make a Mental Health institution. The place is actually built of different materials from the ordinary house. The doorframes, the bathrooms, the cupboards are all of steel. There are protective frames on the windows. It is an entirely abnormal environment and produces abnormal behaviour.

There is nothing homelike about a ward, largely as a result of pressure of numbers. The most noticeable difference is one of size and scale – a bedroom with forty beds, a dayroom for forty children. There is little of the division of space by use found in a home. The small kitchen is used only for washing dishes and is never entered by the children. The playroom is also a dining-room, an occasional bedroom, and a changing-room. There is a bathroom but because of staff pressures a large amount of nappy-changing takes place in both the other areas. Lack of differentiation in room use is probably the explanation for some of the socially inappropriate behaviour shown by the children in that they have never been taught that certain activities are usually confined to the bathroom. The numbers in the ward mean that any ward is likely to contain children of widely differing behaviour and levels of functioning. With our present shortage of staff it is always the lowest common denominator of ability and behaviour that will be catered for.

Such a large community worries continually about the risk of cross-infection. At worst this results in shiny white lino floors, shiny white lino walls, enamelled iron beds and cots, white laminex tables and drab vinyl covered chairs with metal legs. Furniture is restricted to these basics, and twin bugbears of neatness and economy dictate absolute uniformity. There are no armchairs, no rugs, no fabrics where a child might reach them. The polished floors are a hazard for children learning to walk, and it is easier for children to skate on their bottoms than to crawl. Respect for personal possessions cannot be taught because there are no personal possessions. No place is provided for a child to keep private treasures. The design of the bathrooms and their fixtures makes toilet training and the teaching of self-help skills difficult.

The lack of fabric to absorb noise, and the vastness and height of rooms aggravate further the noise problems to be expected from any room of forty children. As at a loud party, the noise level spirals upward as each person tries to outvoice the clamour. It is difficult to bring home the extent of the problem to anyone who has not himself experienced it. The noise level obviously distresses some of the children, and is probably responsible for some disturbed behaviour; it certainly has a bad effect on the staff.

The children have no opportunity to participate in food shopping, preparation or cooking; they never see the food they eat before it appears in stainless steel trolleys. There is no opportunity for a child to choose what he will eat, how much he will eat, or even if he will have a drink with his meal. (Drinks are given at 6 a.m., 10 a.m., 2 p.m. and 6 p.m.)

There are strong pressures on the staff to ensure that meals are eaten quickly. This means that relatively few children feed themselves, because it is quicker for the staff to feed them than to teach them. Those children who do feed themselves are served cut food for speed. They eat from bowls with spoons, drink from mugs, and never see a knife, a fork, a plate or a cup and saucer. They never see adults eat and therefore have no idea of what constitutes acceptable meal-time behaviour.

The children who cannot eat by themselves are served mashed or vitamized food to make feeding quicker. They therefore do not experience different tastes and textures. More importantly, they have no chance to chew. Lack of this exercise means that the acquisition of speech will be more difficult. Lack of solid food is also the major cause of the extremely high incidence of gum disease in the hospital. Gum disease affects the children's general health and is incurable except by extracting teeth. Lack of teeth, of course, also makes speech acquisition difficult and any speech acquired less distinct than it would be otherwise. Once teeth are extracted the children are condemned to a diet of mush for the rest of their lives. A diet of mush results in constipation, which both makes the children uncomfortable and involves an enormous wastage of valuable staff time rectifying the situation.

Dietary deficiencies are a problem. Few of the children ever have raw fruit or vegetables. The dietician of necessity prescribes average quantities of food and leaves to the ward staff the task of re-distributing this according to individual needs. In practice, unfortunately, this usually means that all children get identical servings. While the food is chosen to provide a balanced diet, the processing it undergoes ensures that a high percentage of the volatile nutrients are lost. Kitchen routines result in food being prepared some hours before it is needed and being kept warm in heated trolleys. This destroys much of the vitamin content and the conditions are ideal for the multiplication of bacteria. Vitamin deficiencies increase the children's already high susceptibility to nose and chest infections. These infections reduce the level at which the child functions educationally as well as producing cases of conductive deafness which often go undiagnosed in the institutional environment.

Because I was trying to keep to those problems that were common to all the large institutions, I did not tell the Premier's Committee about the peculiar way St Nicholas children were fed. Children, even children who could sit up, were generally laid down to be fed. Their heads would rest in the nurse's lap, and their bodies would lie across another chair placed in front of her knees. This meant children were being fed with their heads tilted right back, a method called, for obvious reasons, 'bird feeding': gravity drops the food straight to the back of the throat, and there is no chance to chew. Children were encouraged not to shut their mouths – a second mouthful immediately followed the first. I have filmed a nurse feeding a child: food is piling high on his face because he is unable to swallow it at the rate the nurse spoons it in. It must have been terrifying. In that position you have very little control over your swallowing, and it is easy to choke. In 1975 each nurse had ten children to feed in an hour, and everything had to be sacrificed to speed. Each nurse now has only five or six children, and the pressure is reduced, but the feeding methods are still similar. How the nurses ever managed to care for ten children, all as dependent as babies, I shall never know.

The provision of clothes reflected the depersonalizing effect of institutions.

Clothes arrive in the ward in sacks and trolleys. The children miss out on the experiences of shopping for clothes and seeing them washed and ironed. As well as this immediate deprivation, the fact that these services are carried out in bulk at one remove from the children they are intended to serve has further drawbacks; the type of clothing provided is dictated by the extreme harshness of the bulk laundering methods used, and the economics of bulk ordering result in the lack of a suitably large range of sizes. There are four basic sets of clothing – boy's summer, boy's winter, girl's summer, girl's winter. There is limited variation in size and colour and none at all in fabric or style. Such everyday items of clothing as cardigans, pyjamas and skirts do not exist for the children. The clothes being specially made for the institution brand the children when they do go into the outside world. (Clothes probably also affect staff attitudes to the children. If a staff member has a favourite the first sign of this is that the child is dressed in non-regulation clothes, thus giving it a more normal appearance.) Only three sizes of clothing – small, medium, and large – are available for a population aged from 1 to 17. (The babies are generally provided with baby clothes – mainly donated.) At the best of times only a few children fit their clothes. At the worst of times the linen-room is unable, because of problems with the central laundry, to supply clothes in the sizes requested by the wards, and children are dressed in sizes so grotesquely inappropriate as to constitute an additional physical handicap. Most of the people the children see are in uniform, which again limits their chances of seeing other kinds of clothes and feeling different kinds of fabrics. Because of staff shortages children are not encouraged to dress themselves – here, again, it is easier to do it for them than to teach them. This not only means that the child can't dress himself but also that he has lost one of the most basic opportunities for finding out about his own body – concepts like left and right, back and front.

Things have improved a bit since then. For one thing, many of the children have turned sixteen and have started getting the invalid pension. Those on pensions are gradually accumulating private wardrobes, and some non-government clothing has been bought with money from the child endowment fund. But there have been no basic changes. My submission went on to say:

St Nicholas, like any other large institution, tends to get out of touch with the needs of the people it is meant to serve. This is partly because care is provided within narrow specializations; instead of a mother and a father the children have nurses, maids, cleaners, cooks, boiler-attendants, drivers and gardeners. Each of these has his own concept of his job and if he is not directly involved in handling children the children may play no part in this concept. The gardener, for example, opposes children playing with paints on the lawn because it makes the grass dirty. More seriously, the work times established by several of the staff unions bear no relation to the real needs of a residential institution. The timetable that results bears no relation to the timetable followed by normal children. St Nicholas children have lunch at 11.30 and their evening meal at 3.30, after which there is a sixteen-hour wait for breakfast at 7.45. All the children's activities have, therefore, to be so arranged that the children will be back in the wards at 3.30; they miss the most appropriate TV programmes, as these come on when they are eating or being got ready for bed, their day is absurdly shortened, and the scope for any activities outside the ward is very much reduced. As in so many matters, arrangements cater for the lowest common denominator. St Nicholas has in its wards some very young children, and it is these who suffer least from being put to bed with the light out at five o'clock. Seventeen-year-olds in the same ward are rather worse off.

The professional staff are also affected by the constraints of the institution. Children in care tend not to be given the rigorous checks on physical condition that would probably be given children at home. A child with eczema, for example, will not be checked for food allergies, though his hands may be bandaged to stop him scratching – which also, of course, bars him from any productive activity. Once a child has been admitted with a diagnosis of severe retardation there is a tendency to assume that everything that needs to be said has been said, and doctors may be unwilling to arrange for such things as the hearing tests which normal children (who have far less chance of being deaf) have as a matter of course in their school medical examinations; it does not seem to occur to them that the discovery of deafness in a young child might cast doubt on the original diagnosis of severe retardation... For the hospital as a whole the size of the population means that there is a tendency to take services in to the child rather than taking the child out to the service. Hair-cuts, dentists, doctors, new clothes and such entertainment as there is are all provided within the compound. This means that the children miss out on a lot of valuable social experiences, chances of meeting normal people and experiencing life in the normal world.

The pressures of routine exert themselves right down the line. The daily routine is as unvarying as the food and the clothes. A child due to sit on the toilet at a certain time sits there regardless of whether it was dirty ten minutes previously. All children are put to bed at the same time, a whole ward's nappies are changed at once. Care is reduced to the lowest common denominator, not because of the decisions of individual staff but because of the pressures of the institution. No matter how absurd the degree of regimentation, the staff will be able to find justification for any particular instance. The physically handicapped children who lie on rubber mats in the dayroom are always laid in exactly the same position on exactly the same mat. As the children are paralysed their only chance of seeing the other children in the ward or to view the ward from a different angle would be to have their positions changed frequently. The staff explain the present practice by saying 'It's so we know where they are.'

To this you have to add the factors peculiar to St Nicholas at that time: a largely untrained staff, most of whom had a poor command of English; vast overcrowding and extreme understaffing; buildings totally unsuited to their functions (two of the wards had no toilets); no toys, almost no decorations, and children spending their entire lives lying on their backs because there was no proper seating. Maureen Oswin has movingly documented the intense isolation suffered by handicapped children in similarly deprived institutions in England. In her book *Children in Long Stay Hospitals*, she records that she observed the behaviour of staff and children over a period of eighteen months. She found that each child received an average of five minutes of mothering a day, that is, of playing, talking, and cuddling and an average of an hour's bodily care. The amount of time for the majority of

St Nicholas children who had no physiotherapy would have been similar.

Some things have certainly changed since 1975. There are fewer children now, and the staff ratio is better. There are more activities programmes, and the children go for excursions outside the hospital more frequently. The wards are highly decorated, there are many television sets and record players, and lots of toys.

Meal times are still the same, however, even though the children are five years older, and nineteen-year-olds must still be in their cots by five o'clock. Many children do not leave the ward from week's end to week's end. Most children still have no physiotherapy, no boots, and no wheelchairs. By their nature, the rigidities of hospital life have changed the least.

One other thing has not changed. St Nicholas is still an 'informal' institution. When I first came in 1974 I found that some of the more difficult children were being tied up in a particularly brutal manner: I raised it with the Manager, mentioning the strict limits placed on such restraints by the Mental Health Act. 'Oh, didn't you know?', he said. 'St Nicholas isn't covered by the Act.' For administrative convenience St Nicholas had not been gazetted under the Mental Health Act, which is mainly concerned with the management of psychiatric patients. None of the protections set down in the Act applied to it, and as a government institution it did not have to observe any of the regulations that applied to private nursing homes. (If it had been a private business it would have been closed down for overcrowding.) St Nicholas slipped neatly between two stools.

When I started work at St Nicholas in 1974 I had no idea of the kind of place I was getting into and no idea at all that I would still be there six years later.

ANNIE: I lived in St Nicholas Hospital until I turned eighteen.

Until I was sixteen I was totally unable to communicate with any adult because I am a severely handicapped athetoid. Athetosis is a type of cerebral palsy which results in a lot of uncontrolled movement; as well, in my case, there was an enormous excess of muscle tension. The combination of these difficulties meant that I could not use my hands, walk, or talk intelligibly.

In 1977 I was taught to communicate by using an alphabet board on which I point to letters in order to spell sentences. That is how I wrote my part of this book.

The worst thing for me about going into an institution was the total separation from everything I had known. St Nicholas would not allow parents to leave toys or clothes when they left a child. My rabbit, which I loved dearly, could not come, and neither could the animals we had as pets. The ruthless way in which children were parted from their toys was typical of the system's treatment of children. We upset all their rather puritanical ideas about how children should behave. We were not good patients. We cried because we felt abandoned. The nurses didn't know what to do; they didn't know we could feel anguish. The institution had no tally book for broken hearts.

Nurses were discouraged from cuddling children. A crying child needed to be punished for its own good, so it would learn to accept the absence of affection and be happy. Punishment consisted of locking the crying child in a small dark store room. The hospital defined a happy child as a quiet child. Silence was not only golden but sullen; the nurses never saw the looks we gave them when a child was put away.

The doctors were no better. They went home at night, when the crying was worst.

Remembering home was easier when you were in your cot with no toys, no games, no stories and no tucking in. We didn't want to be kissed goodnight – that would have been unbearably distressing – but it would have been nice if someone had shown some sign that they would be glad to see us in the morning.

Talking about shit filled an enormous part of the nurses' days. They spoke only a limited form of English, so the words they used were usually those used as abuse in polite society. You used to hold off shitting until you just about burst rather than suffer the abuse. We could not take ourselves to the toilets even if there had been toilets, so we were all in nappies.

If you did not use your bowels you would have a suppository rammed in. This was recognized by the authorities, who had provided a tome in which all movements were recorded for posterity. It was called the Bowel Book. This caused no end of problems, because failure to score resulted automatically in laxatives. One day missed meant Duralax tablets; two, suppositories; three, an enema. You had no say at all. Some nurses never marked the book, so totally unnecessary suppositories were frequently given. If you had a shit after being given a suppository you still had to listen to remarks about your odour and messiness. Instead of giving laxatives at night when they would cause the least embarrassment, they were always given at breakfast or lunch, ensuring a totally ruined morning or afternoon. This would not have mattered once in a while, but some of us were being dosed every second day.

Still, we thought we would be going home. Perhaps we were going to be cured. Little did we know! St Nicholas only has 'hospital' in its title because it occupies the old Children's Hospital buildings. Of course, these were available for us only because they had been condemned as unsafe and inappropriate for children. Less medical care was given than we had at home. Laughter was the only medicine apart from laxatives and anticonvulsants.

Humour was discouraged because laughter was confused

with epilepsy and treated by injecting Valium or paraldehyde. The nurses had never seen physically handicapped people before and had no idea which responses we shared with normal kids and which were significant indications of distress requiring intervention.

Jittery nurses often thought we were frail and used to keep us in bed until the temperature had hit eighty. This resulted in even those children who had no physical handicap becoming wasted and pale. For the spastics, lying flat was disastrous. Their spasm became worse lying flat than sitting, reduced their ability to speak clearly, blocked gesturing, and usually removed any means of interaction. We were each marooned in our private cage. Vitality ebbed. We became prey to infections, which proved to the nurses that they were right to keep us in bed. The ultimate irony was that outsiders used to commend the nurses for treating us so well.

Despite this I was very attached to some of the nurses from the beginning. I think that some did marvellous work to cope with the numbers of kids in their groups and still be affectionate to us. They treated us like babies, but some treated us like nice babies.

I was very fond of the night nurse on Ward 4. She was never flustered and was always even-handed in the way she dealt with us. You always got good treatment regardless of whether you responded or not.

We took some time to realize that we were not being treated. You expect a hospital to discharge patients other than in coffins. Some kids did come for temporary stays; funnily enough they frequently died. Usually children who visited knew when they were leaving. This meant that they did not become part of the ward and they took a superior attitude to us long-term residents. (As usual, I am talking about those who could communicate – most could not.) We tried not to hate them. It was difficult. Not only were they going home but they also got more than their fair share of attention. The nurses used to make a fuss of them and compare us unfavourably to them. The nurses felt no responsibility if we were skinny, sickly and sullen.

We had ways of communicating between ourselves. Usually we tried to cheer up any short-stay kids by pointing out how much better their state was than ours. We felt that nowhere could be as dreadful as St Nicholas; however, it seemed that the outside had its problems too. Most short-stay kids we saw were very physically handicapped. Those who spoke were generally unhappy because no one understood them, and they had no one to talk to. At least we had each other. Sometimes kids wanted to help us, but telling others was impossible for them too.

Dying was dependent on the way you felt. Jobs in mental hospitals do not attract the best doctors, and there was no supervision. The patients could not complain. If you wanted to die you had every opportunity. Many short-stay kids took their chance. Death never appealed to me; I wanted revenge. Now that does not seem to matter. What is important is stopping other kids going through what we went through. Time was when the strongest emotion I felt was hate, and hate makes you strong. Tender emotions were dangerously softening. Implacable hatred of the whole world which hunted handicapped children into middens like St Nicholas twisted my relationships with people for years.

Deceiving yourself was the hospital pastime. You imagined you talked perfectly and that you would be taken out for ever. You imagined waking up cured. You never took your condition seriously; it was never as important to you as it was to others. We had never walked; it did not look like we ever would. It was something we had grown up knowing. For busting out of confinement, speech seemed more desirable. We knew there were kids in St Nicholas who could walk, but none who could talk properly. All our imaginings depended for their fulfilment on speech.

Chapter Two

Because St Nicholas was so completely isolated from all the educational facilities which dealt with physically handicapped children, everybody who worked there took it for granted that the children were retarded. Most of the visitors came to visit retarded children, not physically handicapped children, and the children who were intelligent did not realize that there were other similarly handicapped but intelligent children who had been given ways of communicating with normal people. As Annie said, 'We thought we were the only ones.' The implications of this are horrible. The intelligent children must have thought they were irrevocably confined inside their bodies, and because they could not find a way of telling normal people they were intelligent, there would be no way any adults would ever discover it for themselves.

By chance I was to discover it. It took immense good luck. It also took three years.

I first met Annie early in 1974 when I was being taken around the wards by one of the assistant matrons. Annie was on the floor in the Ward 4 playroom. She was lying on her side. The nature of her problem meant that she could not lie on her back. Her legs were bent backward, her head and neck were extended backward, and her arms were pushed out behind her. She was shaped like a bow, with her arms as the bowstring almost touching her heels. I had never seen a child in such a position before. Her tongue was going in and out non-stop, and she was incredibly, unbelievably thin. She was about 100 centimetres long. You could see the outlines of her muscles, and her face was like a skull. Her eyes looked large in her face and stared brightly from among a net of laughter lines. Her mouth stretched in a grin when I said 'Hello', and you could see the muscles in her cheek move. The grin heightened her resemblance to a skull.

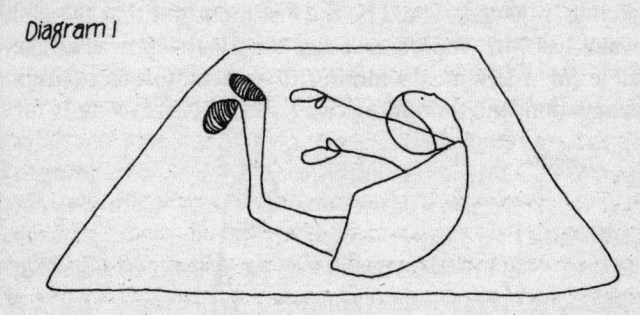

Diagram 1

Very tactlessly I asked the sister who that was and what was wrong with her. I was told that this was Annie. She was thirteen, and she had an enormous muscular spasm which was getting worse and worse. She was getting more and more difficult to feed, I was told, and in another six months her heels would touch her head and she would die. This was said in front of Annie.

The staff at St Nicholas were used to seeing children die. About a hundred and fifty children have died there. Staff members did not like seeing children they were attached to die, and they did not like seeing children die in pain, but when they looked ahead and saw death coming for a child they did not necessarily take any steps to prevent it. Given the kind of life the children were leading, it was defensible, but I was new to the area, and I was not used to a child's death being accepted in this way.

Annie's spasm was so bad by 1974 that she could not sit in any of the chairs available at St Nicholas, and there was a tendency for her to be fed in the most extraordinary position. This meant that all her weight was being taken by her neck, which made it extremely difficult for her to swallow and exacerbated the tongue-thrust, which made it more likely that she would accidentally push back a mouthful of food. At this time the nurses had ten children to feed in an hour. In the circumstances, the first mouthful of food a child 'rejected' would be the last mouthful that the child was given. In Annie's case her tongue-thrust was responsible for many meals coming to a premature conclusion. Starvation, and therefore death, was never far away.

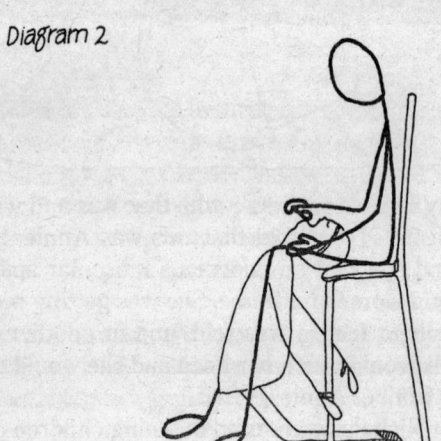

Diagram 2

Annie would have had only tenuous contact with many of the children who died, but she would have heard their deaths talked about by the staff. Some of the children who died were her friends; she knew them very well indeed. At St Nicholas children die publicly in the wards. If it is known that a child is near death a screen will probably be put around the cot, but death often comes without that preparation.

More deaths occur in the so-called sick ward, where the frailer children live, than in the other wards, and Annie lived in that ward for some time. There is no doubt that she would have had considerable contact with death and dying.

When a child dies no attempt is made to keep it from the other children or to break it to them clearly and gently. Instead, the children who can not see or hear the death are likely to find out about it when the staff are hunting around for a shroud of the right size and are calling across the ward to arrange supplies of cotton-wool for the laying out. Children in the other wards hear it on the grapevine. The staff talk about it, and if they only use a nickname or a part of a name the children have to work out for themselves who has died.

In my position as administrative assistant to the Training Officer one of my duties was to arrange practical work experience for student teachers. I set up arrangements to visit schools and training centres around Melbourne, and I also had to run a programme in which the students would work with some of the children. That involved looking through the wards.

Before my playgroups began, the children chosen for the students had been the most physically able. It was assumed that they would also be the most able intellectually. This surprised me. Although I did not know any of the children, my work at the Spastic Centre had shown me that if you are dealing with children with cerebral palsy you cannot assume anything from the severity of their physical handicap. Statistics certainly showed that on average the more severe the physical handicap the more severe the mental handicap, but that was an average, and it did not say anything about any particular child. Furthermore, all the literature referred frequently to people who did not fit into the overall trend, whose physical handicaps were severe but who were intellectually above average.

Because I felt it was unfair to choose only children who were physically able (unfair both to the more handicapped children in the wards and to any physically handicapped children the students would be working with in the future), I set out to select a group of 'brighter' but very physically handicapped children. Jean Vant, my boss, was happy to give her permission.

I went around the wards asking children to perform simple acts to try to assess their verbal comprehension. None of the children could speak, and it was obviously inappropriate to ask them to perform physical tests. They had experienced very little that they could be tested on. I went about it in this way. I would look at Leonie, for example, getting the name from the end of the cot, and say, 'Is your name Mark?' The child would look at me in a puzzled kind of a way. 'Is your name Leonie?' If that got a big beaming smile, the chances were that Leonie recognized her name. 'Can you blink your eyes, like this?' (I had to show them what I meant). Any child who was able to blink on command was probably able to understand spoken language.

All this was based only on probabilities. It was essential to ask a lot of different kinds of questions, so that eventually the sheer number of questions ruled out the possibility of a child's passing the test by random responses. I used to hold out two objects in my outstretched hands and say, 'Look at the hand I've got the spoon in.' I would do this with a series of objects, moving the nominated objects randomly from hand to hand. 'Can you move one of your hands?' If so, I could ask the child to touch things. I would lean over the cot and tell the child to hit me on the nose; children love hitting people on the nose. Every now and again I got my nose hit. 'Can you stick out your tongue?', I asked.

All these questions were designed to see how much

language the children understood. I was not trying to do an exhaustive assessment of all the children in the hospital. I was trying to find eight very physically handicapped children who had good language comprehension. I did not care how many children I missed as long as I found eight, so anyone who was not feeling well, or did not like my face, or was deaf and did not respond simply missed out. It was a matter of whipping around a hundred and sixty children very quickly.

Annie did perfectly on the simple comprehension tests I gave her and was one of the eight children I chose for my group. Of those eight, two turned out to have been chosen wrongly: their intellectual level was not up to that of the other children in the group, although their motor skills were greater and had misled me. Two of the children in the group have since died. The other four – Annie, Mark, Angela, and Lesley – I worked with until May 1980. They were the nucleus of the group that became known as the Beanbaggers. The group expanded during my years at St Nicholas as I got to know the children in the wards better and found more who belonged in it. Some children stayed in the Beanbaggers only long enough for me to decide I had been wrong about them (by that time I had set up other groups, and demotion did not mean losing everything).

In the beginning I thought of the Beanbaggers only as a playgroup. When it started to meet the student teachers provided the labour and I acted as supervisor. In the group the more handicapped children did the same kinds of things as the comparatively physically able. Some of the more energetic activities were obviously impossible, but the point of the exercise was to make it clear to the students that it was possible to do ordinary pre-school activities with all children regardless of their physical handicaps.

We were working on the basis that the highest mental age we were likely to find at St Nicholas was about three or four. We knew that we were dealing with children who had missed out on almost all ordinary experiences. Even the children with more motor skills had had very little opportunity for guided constructive play, and the very physically handicapped children had not had an opportunity to play at all since they had come into the hospital.

The group met once a week during 1974. As the students only did practical work for the first two terms, it was scheduled to finish in August. But I could not bear to disband the group. My boss, who was very flexible and very keen to do more for the children in the hospital, was prepared to allow me to continue to run it with whatever help I could get. The more mobile children were now catered for by a kindergarten programme that had been started earlier in the year on the initiative of the physiotherapist and which operated for one day a week with two staff. The end of the programme was not as hard on them, and I went on working with the physically handicapped group.

One of the first things I did with the Beanbaggers in 1974 was to try to establish some kind of yes/no response for each child. As they could not talk to me, any communication between us was going to depend on my asking them questions and their indicating replies. At the Spastic Centre I had worked with an athetoid girl who had the same kind of tongue-thrust as Annie, and she had indicated yes and no by tongue movements. I suggested to Annie early in 1974 that she might do the same.

I went up to the ward one evening after Annie had been given her dinner and put to bed. I did most of my work with the children then, because I still had my administrative job during the day. I took Annie out to the deserted dayroom and talked to her, sitting on the floor next to her. I explained that I had worked with other children like her and that they had all used yes/no responses, and I told her that if our relationship was going to develop any further she would need to be able to communicate with me. A yes/no response, I suggested, would be helpful. Janet, at the Spastic Centre, had put her tongue back behind her teeth for 'no' and had squeezed her tongue between her lips for 'yes'.

'Do you understand what I've been saying?', I asked.

She held her tongue out with a tremendous grin.

It must have been immensely exciting for Annie, but I should have realized that her answer and that grin were not the responses of a profoundly retarded child. I did not think as deeply as I should have about the speed with which she had acquired the yes/no response or the way in which she had used it. I even told students about the incident afterwards to show them that profoundly retarded children were sometimes able to learn in unexpected ways. But I did not take it the way I should have; I did not take it any further. Poor Annie. She was so happy; she must have thought the world was going to open up for her then.

During the next two or three years she was the most enthusiastic participant in any group's activities, although seating her was a major problem. She could lie on her side in a beanbag with difficulty, but then her head went back and she could not see. She could not sit up in a pusher because she pushed out into an arch. I once carried her across from the ward to the playgroup and ended up with bruises on my arms, not because she had been kicking or struggling but because I had been trying to contain her enormous muscular spasm. I spoke to the medical officer about the spasm and she tried to control it with doses of diazepam (a drug better known by one of its brand names, Valium). Over the next couple of years the dosage was increased until Annie was on 40 milligrams of diazepam a day. That is a lot for a normal adult, and it was a lot more for someone who weighed only 12 or 13 kilograms.

Medication did not diminish her spasm, although together with my efforts at better positioning, it did stop it from getting worse. She could still be fed enough to sustain life, although barely, and she survived.

ANNIE: I was too fearful of dying to appreciate what Rosie's coming could mean. Sister Z said I would die in six months. Until Rosie asked Z to do something about my spasm I did not think anything could be done; all the nurses said that it would get so bad that they would not be able to feed me. It was upsetting to think that it would be starvation that would kill me.

Death lived in the wards at St Nicholas. He was often more friendly than the nurses. Death walked around my cot, but he never felt that my ribs were well enough covered to stand the worms a feed. For much of the time I spent at St Nicholas Death would have accorded me the greatest pleasure by paying me a visit.

Just recollecting life before Rosie came depresses me. Until I saw her talking to kids, I did not know any person who was not handicapped who thought such handicapped people could understand.

Cause and effect was the only belief I had; for example, being tough meant that you would not be popular but would live longer.

ROSIE: 'What do you mean by being tough?'

ANNIE: 'Being tough meant not smiling at baby talk and fighting any liberties taken with your body.'

ROSIE: 'What kind of liberties?'

ANNIE: 'Tickling, attempts at force-feeding, etc.'

ROSIE: 'What made you think that being tough made you live longer? Didn't the favourites get better treatment?

ANNIE: 'I think that being a pet softened the spirit so that when you stopped being a favourite you lost the will to live.'

ROSIE: 'Were you ever a pet?'

ANNIE: 'Yes.'

ROSIE: 'How come you survived?'

ANNIE: 'I was a pet when I knew the risks and could guard against them.'

ROSIE: 'About how old were you when you were a pet?'

ANNIE: 'Eight.'

ROSIE: 'How were you able to guard yourself against the risks?

ANNIE: 'By being careful not to become dependent on any one person.'

ROSIE: 'Why did you stop being a pet?'

ANNIE: 'Staff changes. Being dropped still upset me terribly, so much so that I vowed never to allow myself to become fond of any staff again. Children could be trusted, but not adults.'

When Rosie suggested I use my tongue for yes and no I was excited by the possibilities. For the first time I was able to choose some of the things that happened to me. Until Rosie came, no one tried to check if we understood anything. I was extremely relieved that someone did look beyond our bodies. It meant that there were people who did not believe that physical skills determined intellectual development.

I was so happy. Meeting the rest of the kids was enough for a start. I had known some of them before I went to Ward 4, but I was not even sure that they were still alive. Forming friendships at St Nicholas was a chancy business because if you were moved you would never revisit your old ward. Kids were placed according to staff wishes, so friendships could be broken for ever by the stroke of a pen.

Chapter Three

I was becoming progressively more involved in the life of the wards, largely through the operation of the cash nexus. Setting up the playgroup had meant that we needed a lot more toys and equipment, and I discovered from the Manager that there was a large amount of accumulated money waiting to be spent. Government child endowment payments had been coming in regularly for every child in the hospital, and as nobody except the physiotherapist had ever done anything with the money, I was told that there was about $60 000 in the kitty. The Manager was only too willing for me to spend it.

I worked up gradually. First we got the equipment for the playgroup: beanbag chairs (most of the children could not sit in anything else), and baby buggies and pushers, because it had become clear that transport was a problem. Life in St Nicholas had left the children small for their age, which meant that they fitted comfortably into baby buggies.

When the equipment was improved, I went around trying to brighten the wards. At first I met with a lot of resistance. Many of the staff had been there for years, and they saw the place as a hospital, not a home. They felt that it should be run on the medical model, and posters were frowned upon because they collected germs and dust. The same was true for mobiles and toys. Toys were for special occasions.

I remember putting up my first posters of a puppy, a kitten

and a duckling: three or four posters in one ward. The Assistant Matron tore them down saying they were totally inappropriate. Fortunately there were two New Zealand nurses at St Nicholas who had very different ideas, and they gave me my opportunity. The Assistant Matron went on holidays, the New Zealanders encouraged me, and gradually a bit of competition emerged among the younger staff. 'You're getting posters for her ward,' they would say, 'why not for mine?'

I put up a mobile and primed the next group of visitors to comment favourably on it to Matron; Matron ordered me to put up more mobiles immediately. I was really pleased. I got the students to make more mobiles to hang from the ceilings of the hospital's huge rooms. Gradually more posters were put up, and toys were attached to the children's cots so they had something to touch. A cassette recorder was bought for each ward so that there would be music. I spent my time running around from ward to ward swapping posters about; we did not have nearly enough, and the ones we had needed to be changed often to stimulate the children. As the children were not taken outside the hospital we had to vary the atmosphere inside as much as we could. I stuck tactile things along the bottom of the walls to give the children variety of touch, I changed cassettes from ward to ward, and I tried to convince the administration that it would be a good thing to buy a colour television set for each ward. I wrote a submission which said:

Some of our children have quite a good perception of what happens on TV and can cope with a black and white picture. If they had a normal existence there would be no reason for them to have a colour television; however, as things are it is their only view of life outside the ward. If you were to read a story to this group of children you would see very quickly how limited their world is and how colour television could expand it. For example, convention in stories and illustrations dictates that water is blue. If the only water you've seen comes out of a tap what colour is that water? What does 'blue' mean to such a child?

The authorities were afraid that the staff would sit and watch television instead of doing their jobs, which they sometimes did; but nonetheless television was vital for these children.

During that year I talked a lot to my friends about how seldom the children went out of the hospital, and one of them contacted a social involvement group at the University of Melbourne, which was nearby. The group arranged to send volunteers to the hospital once a week, and I arranged for the children to be taken out for walks. It was so unheard of that I had to send letters to all the parents asking them for permission to take their children outside the hospital grounds.

Towards the end of 1974 I was thinking again of applying for other courses. My job as assistant to the Training Officer was ending because the course structure had been altered. The Manager and Superintendent, however, asked me if I would stay on and work full-time with the children. They wanted me to develop a programme of activities, keep up the effort to provide a more stimulating environment in the wards, and give the children more chances to get outside. I agreed happily. In 1975 I became the first full-time person in charge of activities at the hospital. I was still on the books as a ward assistant: the administration made efforts to have me reclassified, but there was no position in the Mental Health Authority for anyone who did not fit its two categories of nurse or therapist.

In my new job and with all this encouragement I started spending money like a drunken sailor. Part-time workers could be hired as play-leaders out of the government's child endowment money, so we hired some. A few were trained teachers looking for part-time work, but most were university students whom I trained on the job. We moved into some of the rooms that the student teachers had evacuated, and for the first time the children had a place to call their own outside the ward.

All these were fairly minor changes, and I could see that major changes were necessary if the children were to have reasonable lives. But the changes had to be made at a higher level. The Premier of Victoria had set up a committee to inquire into all aspects of care and education for the retarded, and in May 1975 I gave the committee a paper entitled 'The Handicapping Effect of our Present System of Care for Mentally Handicapped Children, and a Possible Remedy'. I spoke about my submission and showed a videotape of St Nicholas at a public hearing on 10 November 1975, and next day's newspapers gave what I had said wide coverage. The meal times were commented on particularly. An editorial in the *Age* was headed 'Bedtime at St Nicholas' and said in part, 'It is surely scandalous that children are given their evening meal at 3.30 and put to bed at four . . .' The *Herald*'s editorial, 'Rules are Rigid – Children Suffer' said that my evidence 'will shock those who thought that such an approach passed with pre-Dickensian days . . . children are put to bed "for the night" at four in the afternoon, and endure a sixteen-hour gap from "dinner" to breakfast.'

It says something about the power of the press and the bureaucracy that the meal times remain the same now as they were before the editorials.

In any case, my name was mud at St Nicholas. The nurses were furious. They thought that they were being criticized, which was not what I had intended. Most Australians will remember something else that happened on 11 November 1975, and what was shaping up as a thorough-going scandal that would throw St Nicholas wide open and reveal a lot of skeletons in the closets was eclipsed by the sacking of the Prime Minister by the Queen's representative, the Governor-General, Sir John Kerr. In retrospect, this overshadowing may have been a good thing. Certainly it was for Annie. If St Nicholas had been cleaned up then, I would have left feeling smug, Annie would have been left behind, and she would probably now be dead.

The Premier's Committee was not able to do anything about the problems at St Nicholas, and in 1976 I took the question of the children's meal hours to Victoria's Ombudsman. The Ombudsman had been dealing with some complaints from prisoners at Pentridge, Melbourne's maximum security prison, and one that he found to be justified was that it was an unreasonable hardship for the prisoners to have their evening meal at 3.30 p.m. and their breakfast at 7.30 in the morning. I wrote him a short note saying that if this was tough on prisoners, was it not also tough on the handicapped children in state institutions who had the same meal times? I was misguided enough to sign it. He took it to the Mental Health Authority officials and asked if they had heard of Rosemary Crossley. He made an inquiry, of sorts, and found that it was not an unreasonable hardship for the children.

I have no evidence that the early bed-time interferes with the digestion of the evening meal. I accept that many children do become distressed in the mornings, not because they are hungry but, as the Superintendent states, more likely because of boredom.

I do not think that it can be said that the present time at which the evening meals are served to children at St Nicholas Hospital constitutes an unreasonable hardship for them . . .

We did get one big boost in 1976: for the first time the Department of Education sent staff into St Nicholas. I had already made contact with St Paul's School for the Blind and the Monnington Special Education Centre for Deaf/Blind Children. When I first came to St Nicholas it had been the presence of deaf and blind children which had horrified me most. There is no way to assess the intellectual capacity of a child who is both deaf and blind without training the child to communicate. No attempt had been made to do this with these 'retarded', and deaf and blind children. By 1976 we also had a few children going to 'school' at various outside centres for a few days a week, but the arrival of people from the Department of Education was a big step forward. From the beginning of second term we had one full-time trained teacher, one part-time teacher and six or seven teacher aides. Their arrival took some of the pressure off me, because up to that time I had been responsible for the education of a hundred and sixty children. I saw from forty to sixty children a week, and the play-leaders saw another thirty, but that meant that seventy children still missed out on any sort of education. I had tried to include them by visiting the wards and endeavouring to make the general environment more stimulating. However, even the children we were working with only came to us for a few hours each week. There was an enormous amount more to be done, and the arrival of the teachers gave us a chance to get on with it.

In 1976 I also began a part-time course for the Diploma of Education. I had expected to leave St Nicholas that year, and I was only staying on so that the teachers could settle in. I felt that I could not go until someone came to replace me, and I knew that if I left the hospital the Mental Health Authority would not replace me; nobody else would have been hired to do the job I was doing. Because of this I decided that a part-time training course was preferable to a full-time one, and the quickest course available was the Primary Diploma of Education at the Melbourne State College. I arranged to do a large proportion of the course in the area of special education, which dealt with retarded and handicapped children.

I was still working with the Beanbaggers, my 'bright' physically handicapped group. By the end of 1976 there were ten of them coming to playgroup one or two afternoons a week, and I was still offering them what was basically a pre-school programme.

The children ranged in age from ten to fifteen, but their lack of experience meant that there were enormous gaps to be filled. We had the ordinary pre-school activities: sand and water-play, finger-painting, play-dough, adapted as necessary to the handicaps of the children. We cooked, grew plants, staged plays, and we wrote books, all the standard things.

Every session with the children included a story, and the stories gradually grew more sophisticated as the children's concentration increased. We read most of the Picture Puffins and gradually started extending beyond them. We had a Wombles craze that lasted for quite a while, using puppets, posters and records.

I read the children a lot of books from reading schemes designed for slow or retarded readers; there were a number of very good schemes designed for teenagers that had simple stories about everyday life. I talked non-stop throughout all the sessions because the ward staff often failed to talk to the children. I emphasized the meaning of words, and whenever possible I made them concrete. I believe that there are a lot of things we only really understand by experiencing them, and with their physical handicaps the children had not been able to experience very much. I spent my time lifting children on tables, dragging them through tunnels, and so on. All the basic shape, colour and number words were introduced and highlighted. There was a lot of listening work, and we played sound matching games of various types. We used the *Sesame Street* records for background music, playing the same songs session after session: the ABC song, a shape song ('There's a square out there'), counting songs, and a song about parts of the body. There was a lot to do in that area because the children's knowledge of their own bodies was limited by their handicaps. For example, we had 'Get to know your feet' sessions: I would have bowls containing different things, say, iced water, mud, and hot soapy water. I would dip every child's foot into each bowl in turn and talk about the sensations. When I dried their feet I would play with their toes.

Aware that the children had never had an opportunity in the wards to choose things, I arranged to have two kinds of drinks available so that they could choose between them by looking at or pointing to the one they wanted. I also tried to expand their acquaintance with food and drink. Coffee and fresh fruit were two new tastes introduced, for example. Once I was sure all the children knew how to choose I could use this ability to test concepts. To get away from the very limited range of eating utensils used in the wards (mugs, bowls and teaspoons), I bought a picnic set with cups, saucers, and plates in four colours. Before I gave out the drinks I distributed a saucer to each child and then brought around a tray of cups, asking them to choose the one that matched their saucer. I could test their ability to recognize other attributes in the same way, and we eventually started playing games using these skills.

It was all very elementary, and I know now that the work was not at an appropriate level, but it was not entirely wasted.

It was not until 1977 that I began to suspect that the Beanbaggers might deserve something more sophisticated than a playgroup.

ANNIE: I rusted away in St Nicholas until Rosemary showed me that some people did know our helpless bodies could contain a mind, even if she did not realize we could be normal. However, just being thought of as animal, not vegetable, was reason for hope. Playgroups were a force not just in building our concepts but in allowing bright kids from every ward to come together. They allowed us to see other children who could communicate. This meant we were not so alone, even if the others were faring no better than us. Before this we were always terrified of being sent to wards where no one could talk. Fun new activities were water play, sand play, finger-painting – teenagers do not enjoy such baby pursuits usually, but you must realize that this kindergarten was the only play or school we had ever had.

Chapter Four

Joey died at the end of 1976. He was one of the original Beanbaggers. I never felt that he liked me very much, and I thought that he died partly because he gave up hope. I sensed that I had failed him in some way. Joey used to make lots of noises, and it was clear that he was trying to talk, but I could not understand anything he said. Perhaps if I had tried harder or been better at understanding abnormal speech patterns, I would have realized his intelligence and that of the other children earlier. When I did it was too late for Joey.

Joey's death made me take a harder look at the conditions of the other children in the group. At the end of 1976 Annie started to go down hill. She became very depressed, stopped participating in the activities of the group, and started losing weight. She weighed only 13 kilograms and did not have much to lose. I thought Annie had some intelligence, but not much, and I knew I could not stand to see another child with some intelligence die in this way in St Nicholas. I decided to see if I could take her home for a weekend. I had given it a lot of thought because it meant involving Chris Borthwick, the man I had lived with for the past eleven years, in my life at St Nicholas. He had already lived through my interminable stories about St Nicholas, but this would be a much more direct involvement, and a long-term one. If you say you will take a child home for a weekend you can't just leave it at one weekend, you have got to be prepared to take the child home regularly. I felt able to do that and so did Chris; I still occasionally visited the children I had taught at Dame Mary Herring years before, and I had kept up contact with some of the children who had left St Nicholas to go to other institutions.

I had to contact Annie's parents to get permission to take her home. Her mother was overjoyed, and she drove down from the country the day after my telephone call to sign the permission form. She was obviously very happy that someone was taking an interest in her daughter. By a stroke of luck she arrived when Annie and the group were in a playroom having an Easter party. Annie's mother was thrilled just to see Annie's finger-paintings on the wall. She said she had been told that Annie would never be able to do anything like that, and she took a bundle of them home to show the family.

I took Annie home for a weekend in the middle of April 1977. She was an unknown quantity, a sixteen-year-old girl with a comprehension perhaps equivalent to that of a normal six-year-old, although I could not be certain of that.

By the time I was ready to leave work on Friday, Annie had already been in bed for two hours. I pulled on some overalls over her nightdress, covered her top with a wind-cheater so she would look reasonably respectable, and packed up several enormous bags of spare clothing and linen. I took a pusher so that Annie would be mobile and called a taxi. I had to nurse Annie on my knee in the taxi – she could not sit on the seat – and I held her up so that she could see out the window, explaining why we stopped at the traffic lights. She was bubbling with happiness.

When we got home I showed Annie around the house. Chris was not there so I put her into the pusher and we set off to the local shops to meet him. Chris had not met Annie before, and when we ran into him he was as embarrassed as she was. After brief introductions he went home and we went around to the shops. It was quite dark by the time we walked back. I realized that it was the first time that Annie would have been outside at night for many years, and I talked to her about the moon and the stars. At home Chris had set out a meal of bread and cheese and delicatessen bits and pieces. Annie had already eaten dinner at the hospital, but she was quite prepared to have a second and even larger meal. She had never had a slice of bread in St Nicholas, let alone pâté, taramasalata or black olives, but she ate them all; she liked the pâté and the taramasalata; the olives were not to her taste.

After dinner we put her to sleep on a mattress in our room. We were not quite sure what to expect, and we wanted to keep an eye on her. She was well behaved but restless.

On Saturday morning we gave her a bath. There could be no more thought of preserving her modesty here than in the hospital, and without Chris's help bathing would have been impossibly dangerous. In St Nicholas the nurses removed any risk of drowning the children by putting them in metal troughs and hosing them down, but we thought that Annie might appreciate something more civilized, and our odd-shaped bath fitted her arched back perfectly.

After a breakfast of porridge we went to the shops again, this time to buy things. As well as getting the weekend's provisions we called in at Woolworths, and I bought Annie a doll and a Little Golden Book. She was very pleased, and I tucked the doll into the pusher beside her. She was so tiny that it did not look out of place at all. At the shops several people spoke to her and she smiled at them.

I had arranged with our next-door neighbour, Sue Jones, to bring her two children – Sally, five, and Jodie, three – to visit us in the afternoon because I thought that the children would be about the same mental age as Annie. When the children saw how handicapped Annie was they were bewildered. She was lying on the floor, because it was uncomfortable for her to sit in the pusher for any length of time, and on the floor all her differences were highlighted. Sally and Jodie had brought a pull-along Lego toy and showed it to her, and Annie liked that, too. She wriggled and laughed and behaved beautifully.

After the Joneses left we took Annie for a walk to the nearby park and playground. She enjoyed watching the children playing, and doing all the things she could not, and Chris gave her a turn on the slide, the swing and the roundabout. We called in to see a friend from Chris's office, who lived in a house next to the park, and begged some afternoon tea. Annie bore with equanimity the idea that dinner was not going to be served at 3.30. After all, she had eaten more breakfast and more lunch than Chris or I had eaten. There were no problems entertaining Annie when we got home again. We did not have television but we brought her into the kitchen and she was able to watch us wash up and prepare dinner.

We had been invited out to lunch on Sunday, and as it was the last few days of an exhibition of American art we wanted to see at the National Gallery we decided to start early and call in there on the way to lunch. I thought that Annie would be happy enough watching the people, and that it would not worry her if we spent an hour or so at the gallery. Annie surprised me. She did not look at the people, she looked at the pictures. I saw her look at the first picture and made some remark to her about it, and after that she looked at every picture, and it was a large collection. She would look at the picture, then turn around – and that was almost all the unaided physical control she could muster – and wait for me to comment on it. We went around the exhibition like this. Some of the other people at the gallery must have thought it was odd to see someone discussing paintings with a child who not only was very obviously handicapped but also looked all of four years old. It was in the lithographic exhibition next door, however, that Annie made her breakthrough. I wheeled her around in front of a lithograph, and she laughed. She had never been one to laugh meaninglessly, and I looked up to see what she was laughing at. It was a Toulouse-Lautrec lithograph of a fat man dancing in a three-piece suit and spats, poised high on his toes, his arms spread wide, very drunk and absolutely ridiculous. Annie was laughing at a black-and-white lithograph. Profoundly retarded people do not have that kind of response.

ANNIE: That first weekend out I was completely overwhelmed by everything. Remember, I had not spent a night out of St Nicholas since the strike [a nurses' strike in 1975], and that had been the only time I had been out overnight in thirteen years. I had no memories of shops or money. In St Nicholas we never saw money, and everything was paid for by government order. Nothing was bought directly from shops, and we never went to any. Lines of shelves filled with food were something I had seen on TV, but I thought they were only for the ads. I did not dream they really existed. It amazed me that people could be trusted not to eat the food in the shops. If I had been able to grab things from the shelves I certainly would have. I couldn't imagine how people could ever choose.

Supper was a taste sensation. I had never tasted food like it. Rosie has a wide interest in food, and it was not until later that I realized that everybody did not eat such a wide variety of foodstuffs.

From my television viewing I knew scenes often took place in baths which were not stainless steel, but I had never seen one before with blue tiles and brass taps. As I was curved, I fitted the triangular shape perfectly and had the only comfortable bath I had ever had. Letting yourself be pampered is lovely. I had not had the chance before.

Possibly the thing I enjoyed most was bed time with stories and games, a diverting change from a patron saint's hospital where there was neither.

The next day I met Chris and Rosie's friends. Taking everything into consideration I was most impressed by the attempts they made to make me feel welcome. Everywhere I went I was treated as a normal child – a child of six, admittedly, but nonetheless normal. It was the first time I'd had that pleasure.

On Sunday we went to the art gallery. Having no previous acquaintance with art I was interested in pictures largely for what they showed, not how they showed it. Basic theory was touched on in the *Civilization* programmes, of which I had seen bits, but I really did not know what I liked. When I saw the Lautrec I laughed because the man looked ridiculous in his elaborate clothes with arms spread and on tiptoe.

I was sure that Rosie must have known I was intelligent. If not, why did she take me to the gallery? From what she has said since I realize she did not suspect I was different. It makes it all the more amazing that I was treated so well.

Chris is tall, dark and hairy. He talks very fast with a stutter that sounds like a machine gun. His ability to read five books at once is amazing. He can't light the fire without reading the paper he is using first. He is insensitive to criticism, and he often drives us crazy by being completely unable to pass any piece of paper with words on it without reading them.

Chris always treated me and the other kids as though we were completely normal. He never had any difficulty talking to us, unlike most people confronted with a mute. Until Chris came to St Nicholas the other kids did not believe me when I told them that there were people other than Rose who would treat them as intelligent.

Chris was the first male I had known who did not find

me ugly or funny. He seemed to ignore my body totally. In no way did he allow any feelings of distaste to show. This I found incredible after men I had known before.

Chris has done more for us than anyone else besides Rosie, despite constant pressure from the Health Commission.

Chapter Five

I spent the next week thinking about two problems: how to give Annie a means of communicating and how to find the time to teach it to her. At this stage I was meant to be doing practical work on literacy for my Diploma of Education, and all the other students were involved in doing remedial work with children who had reading difficulties. Because of my unusual situation at St Nicholas I had obtained permission from the lecturer to do a project with a Down's syndrome child who could not speak. I had been going to try to teach him to communicate using Bliss symbols, a semi-representational ideographic language developed by Charles Bliss to ease international communication, which is frequently used these days with physically handicapped people.

I had not started and I was able to get permission without any difficulty to change the subject of the project to Anne. That solved the time problem, but it left me the problem of what to teach her. I thought that Bliss had three major defects when used as a communications system for handicapped children. The first and most important is shared by all systems that use a fixed vocabulary not chosen by the user. How does the person using the system tell you that they want a word that is not included in the set? Sometimes it is possible to get at the concept by using combinations of already available words. 'Thing which cuts which fits in the pocket' would give you pocket-knife, if you did not think of nail scissors first. But some words, particularly proper names, specific objects, and emotions, are difficult to do in this way. The second difficulty with Bliss symbols is that they are normally arranged in a grid pattern, which is the hardest for a severely handicapped person to use clearly; the finger or hand used for pointing is very likely to land on the line between two symbols, and the number of symbols that a person can use will be limited not by the number they can learn but by the number that can be arranged within their reach. This problem has been solved to some extent in the past few years by the development of electronic scanning devices, but I did not have any of those in 1977. The third problem was that the methods then being used to teach it in the Victorian Education Department involved a lot of time spent memorizing symbols and little time on actual communication. I still thought that Anne was significantly retarded. I certainly did not think that she had anything like normal intelligence. So I did not envisage her ever learning to spell, and I did not really expect that she would ever be able to string together a complex sentence, or indeed any kind of a sentence at all. As I saw it her major need was for a communications system which she could start to use immediately to make her needs known and which would give her the maximum freedom of communication that her supposed intellectual handicap would allow her.

I did not have answers to any of these problems when I decided to work with Annie. One thing was clear, however: there were a number of prerequisites to be met before you could use any communications system, and I had to be sure that Annie fulfilled them. She needed to be able to make a choice according to the instructions she was given and to be able to indicate her choice clearly. She also needed to have the desire to communicate.

On Tuesday 26 April 1977 I took Annie into the ward playroom at about seven in the evening. Before asking her to do anything I talked to her and told her what I was planning to do.

'Annie, I think I can teach you to talk,' I said. 'Not with your mouth, because nobody can do that, but with your hands, by pointing to pictures of things. But before I do that I have to see if you can point.'

Her face lit up and afterwards she worked as if her life depended on it.

I positioned her lying on her side on the floor, not arched backward this time but curved forward so that her arms were brought around in front of her, and her head was pushed forward so she could see what her hands were doing. I had to kneel behind her to maintain her in this position. I just picked up any available objects near me, placed them in front of Annie and asked her to point to the one I named. I started with two objects and steadily increased the number until we had six, which I changed around frequently. No more could fit into the semi-cirle that was within her reach. She pointed consistently and correctly to everything I named. She was completely calm, and her concentration on the task in front of her was intense.

I was so excited that I brought in the ward sister to watch, and in her presence Annie became very excited. Although she still pointed to a number of objects when asked, she started to laugh so much that she mucked one up. After the ward sister had gone, Annie calmed down and once again worked without making an error.

From this session I knew that Annie definitely had the skills she needed if I was to work with her, and I remember walking through the gardens opposite the hospital that night shaking with excitement, racking my brains for some new method to use. It was clear from the evening's work that if Annie could only select one from a range of six a grid system of Bliss symbols was not going to be very useful for her. Here my training in computer programming came into its own, and walking through the gardens I thought of the Venn diagrams used in set theory. They suggested to me a method for communication. This, for example, could be the set for drinks:

Diagram 3

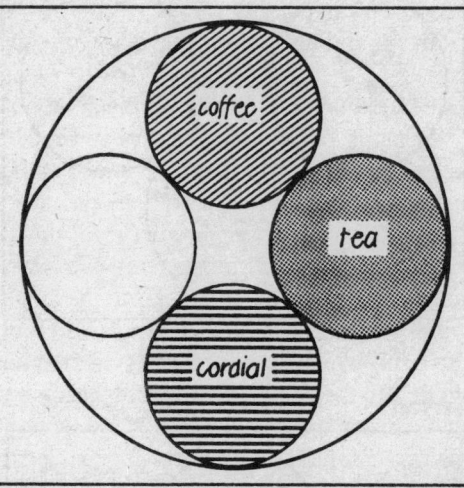

The empty circle would be for 'something else'. If the user wanted milk or water or something that was not named in the set, he had to point to the empty circle, and you could then find out what he was after by asking a series of yes/no questions. Items could be represented in the circles by pictures or symbols or words, depending on who was using it. Communications would eventually involve hierarchies of sets arranged in a book, as in Diagram 4 overleaf.

The numbers in each circle are page numbers. If the person using the system pointed to 'bodily needs', you turned to page 2 and found a set as in Diagram 5 overleaf.

If the person then pointed to 'uncomfortable', you turned to page 6 and found a set as in Diagram 6 overleaf.

Diagram 4

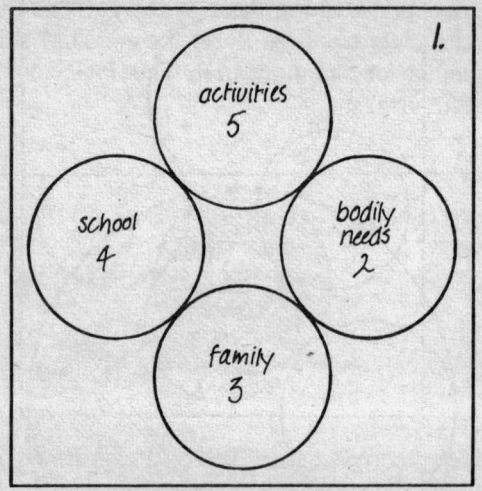

1.
- activities 5
- school 4
- bodily needs 2
- family 3

Diagram 5

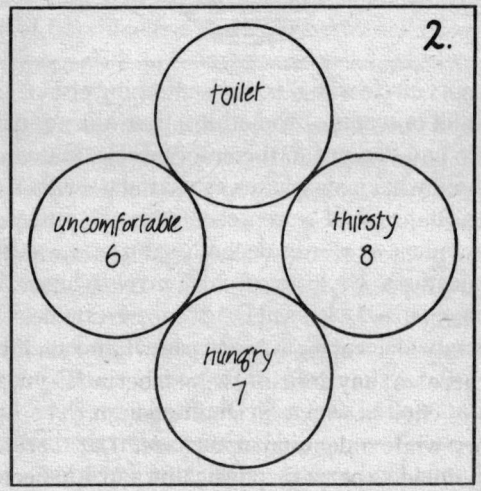

2.
- toilet
- uncomfortable 6
- thirsty 8
- hungry 7

Diagram 6

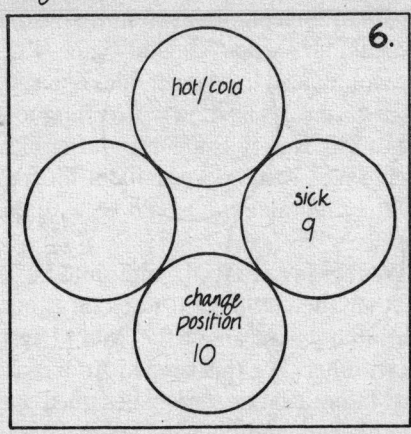

(Diagram showing four circles arranged around a center point. Top circle: "hot/cold". Right circle: "sick 9". Bottom circle: "change position 10". Left circle: unlabeled. Marked "6." in upper right.)

If they then pointed to 'hot/cold' you found out which it was with yes/no questions, using their yes/no responses, whatever they were.

A yes/no question has to be one that can be usefully answered by yes or no. Some people have a tendency to ask a non-vocal child 'Are you hot or cold?' and be surprised when the child does not respond.

It would not be a static language, and you could add other sets whcn you needed them. You could draw them up on the spot as new occasions arose. Because the subsets were at different points of the compass and did not have any common borders, the problem of deciding what the person had pointed to would be minimized. The circles would have to be a good fist size, I decided, to allow ample room for whole-hand pointing. There would be no reason why the user should not be reminded each time what each circle stood for if there was any difficulty remembering them, and every group of choices would be small enough to be held in the memory while a decision was made. The more choices a person could cope with physically and intellectually the

51

fewer sets, and therefore the less pointing, would be needed to reach the end of the communication tree. A person with a 200-word vocabulary who could only cope with three circles at a time would need five hierarchies of circles to cover those 200 words: 3 circles leading to 9 leading to 27 leading to 81 leading to 243. If they could use four circles at a time they would have access to 256 words in the fourth hierarchy of circles, and communication would be both quicker and less arduous.

Next day, Wednesday 27 April, Annie and I had a session to check whether she could point to pictures on request. I was still a bit ambivalent about the kind of system I was going to use with her. For this session Annie sat up in her Baby Buggy Major, a large pusher designed specially for handicapped children, and I pushed her up to a table. This was the best seating available for her at the time, but even so her physical problems were so severe that she could not sit in the buggy in a normal way. Unless you physically held her face to the front, her body would twist around at an angle, and her head would be pushed back and to one side. Although she had been able to point unassisted when she had been lying on the floor with her head and shoulders pushed forward by my knees, once she was sitting in the buggy her shoulders automatically retracted. This made it impossible for her to move her arm, and even if she had managed to get her arm and hand forward she would not have been able to see what her hand was pointing to. In order to get her in a position where she could point to the circles, I had to stand behind her, pushing her head forward with my left hand and supporting her right arm between her shoulder and her elbow with my right hand.

A whole body of literature exists on the techniques of what is called 'facilitation', and there were a number of good reasons for trying the position I chose. I was attempting to counteract the extensor spasm which usually impaired

Anne's control of her movements. The way to achieve this was to have her flexed at the hips with her head and shoulders pushed forward and to provide stimulation for the muscles on the underside of the arm which must be used if the arm is to extend. If I brought Annie's shoulders forward and left her arm unsupported, she would be unable to raise her arm above the table because it would still push back. If you put her arm on the table the enormous pressure with which it pushed down created so much friction that Annie could not move it across the table. Cramp was also a problem and one that is familiar to those working with people who have cerebral palsy. When Annie did manage to move her arm it would often shut up like a rabbit trap: the lower part of her arm would be pressed up against the upper arm or, if her arm had been pushed sideways across her body, it would be pressed across her face, and this meant that she could not reach out to touch anything.

One way of counteracting that was to give stimulation to the extensor muscles that extended the arm while minimizing the amount of stimulation given to the flexors that made it contract; and so I supported her upper arm, which rested on my flat hand. I was acting as a responsive item of furniture, not moving her arm but simply facilitating her own movement. Her pointing was done and is still done by moving her lower arm from the elbow and by moving her hands and fingers. These are movements it would be very difficult to influence by manipulating the upper arm.

I hoped I could use this session to try out this technique of facilitation and to find out a little more about Annie's abilities. To see how well she could point I had assembled a number of photographs of objects around the hospital. They were mounted on pieces of hardboard 150 millimetres square, and the size of the squares meant that only three pictures could fit in a line within Annie's reach. She pointed correctly to the first few objects I named, but it was extremely difficult for her physically, much more so than pointing to objects while she was lying on the floor. We both lost interest in the task after about half an hour. As the difficulties we were having seemed to confirm the fears I had about Bliss symbols, I decided to try the sets I had thought of the night before.

Because Annie was such an unknown quantity, I had to pick an arbitrary level to start from. I decided not to try pictures but to start with a simple system of colour coding. Every time Annie wanted a drink I would produce the set that had 'tea' in the blue circle at the top, 'coffee' in the brown circle on the right, and so on. I wrote names on the coloured circles so I would be able to remember them myself and so it would be easier to explain the system to outsiders; I also hoped that in the long run Annie might be able to learn to recognize a few words if she saw them repeated often enough. Because the system was intended to respond to Annie's needs and not to be imposed on her, I checked to see that she was thirsty and then drew up the circles of the drinks set in front of her, telling her what I was doing. I coloured the circles in, explaining that the blue circle at the top of the diagram was going to be for tea and if she wanted a drink of tea she should point to that circle. I wrote 'tea' on it. The brown circle to the right was going to stand for coffee, and I wrote 'coffee' on it. The red circle at the bottom was for cordial, and I wrote 'cordial' on it. The fourth circle was not coloured in and I did not write anything on it. The blank circle was to stand for 'something else'. She was to point to that one if she wanted a drink that was not tea, coffee, or cordial – milk, for example. I did not go into the concept of the blank circle in any detail because it seemed a bit abstract. I did not think we would be getting to that stage for a couple of months, but for consistency I thought we should have a blank in the set from the start. I went through the circles again, putting Annie's hand on each in turn, saying something like, 'That's where you put your hand if you want tea, on the blue circle', each time. Then I asked Annie what she would like to drink. She pointed clearly to 'coffee'. This had been her favourite drink in the playgroup, so I was not surprised. Just to make sure that it had not been an accident, I moved her hand away from the board and asked her to point to her choice again, and she pointed to 'coffee'. I made her a cup of coffee, and after she had finished I asked her if she would like another cup. 'Yes', she responded, she would, and she chose coffee again.

I said she could choose what we would do next, and I drew up another set of choices. This time the choices were 'walk' (pink circle, to the left), 'music' (yellow circle, at the top), 'paint' (blue circle, to the right), and the empty circle (at the bottom). Annie chose 'walk'; I would have been surprised if she had chosen anything else. The children at St Nicholas have always been positive that they would prefer going out of the hospital to doing even the most enticing activity inside it. Every time Annie made a choice I checked it with her using yes/no responses: 'Is that a walk you want?', 'Does that mean you want a walk?', and I got her to repeat the pointing. I would move her hand completely away from the large circle and say, 'I wasn't quite clear about that – could you point again?' As she had chosen 'walk' I had to draw up another set of circles to see where she wanted to go.

I deliberately drew up all these circles, coloured them in and wrote on them in front of Annie, and I think that this was an important part of the teaching process.

I drew up the set of destinations in exactly the same format as the previous two sets: 'park' (brown circle, at the top), 'shops' (red circle, to the right), 'hospital', which meant the hospital garden (blue circle, at the bottom), and the empty circle (the circle for 'something else', to the left). When I presented her with the sheet of paper and asked her to make her choice she pointed to the empty set. I was astounded.

55

I thought she must have made a mistake. I asked her to point again. Again she pointed to the blank circle. I checked with her using her yes/no responses.

'Is there somewhere else you want to go, somewhere I have not got on the paper?'

'Yes', she responded.

I thought that I had listed all the places within walking distance of St Nicholas. I could not work it out. And then it struck me. When I had drawn the 'park' circle and coloured it in, I had said, 'Park – you know, the park over near the Exhibition Buildings, the park with the lake in it.' As it happens, the park over the road from the hospital is cut in two by the Exhibition Buildings and its associated car parks. One side has a lake, the other side has an adventure playground. I had not meant to make a firm choice of the side with the lake in it, I thought that we would get to the corner and decide which way to go from there.

I said, 'You mean you want to go to the park with the playground in it, do you?'

'Yes!' A big clear 'Yes'.

She might have been thinking that she would get another crack at a slide now. I wrote 'playground' on what had been the empty circle and coloured it pink. I asked Annie to point to where she wanted to go, and she pointed to 'playground'. We went, but I did not give her a go on the slide, because there was too much lifting involved.

I was excited telling Chris about it that evening – excited as much because my system worked as because Annie was doing so well, although I had been surprised and impressed by the way she had used the empty set.

The next day we had a short session to check on Annie's memory for this work. After checking that she wanted a drink I presented the drinks set, without reminding her in any way what the circles stood for. I asked her to point to what she wanted to drink, and she chose 'coffee' without hesitation. While I was making the coffee I asked her to point to the circles for 'tea' and for 'cordial', and she pointed correctly to both. When I asked her what she wanted to do she chose 'walk' again, and for destination she pointed to the circle for 'shops'. I checked with her yes/no responses.

'Do you want to go to the shops?'

'Yes', she indicated.

I asked her to point to where she had been yesterday, and she pointed to 'playground'. I asked her to point again to what it was she wanted to do today, and this time she pointed to 'playground'. I asked her if she had changed her mind – after all, chopping and changing might just mean that she had been pointing randomly – and she gave a sort of yes and no response, moving her hand back and forth between 'shops' and 'playground'.

'Do you want to go to both?', I asked.

She gave a big smile and a definite 'Yes'.

We were short of time, and I told her that she would have to choose one or the other. This time she pointed quite definitely to 'shops' and we went off to the shops, getting her a pair of second-hand boots and a pair of socks, the first she had had since I had known her.

This day's work was even more promising than the last. Remembering the sets without prompting after only one showing was really quite remarkable. The next day was Friday, and Annie came up briefly to show off to some teachers who came each week from Monnington. I told Annie that it would only be a short session – she could choose a drink and meet some people, but there would be no walk because it was nearly lunch time. She turned and looked at the clock! She used the drinks set perfectly adequately in front of the teachers, pointing to 'tea' as the drink she wanted now, and 'coffee' when she was asked what she had had the day before. One doubting Thomas poured a lot of cold water on her achievements and suggested to me that I was moving her arm, intentionally or not. After that, another teacher came in and also wanted to see Annie perform. I asked Annie if she wanted to show off again and got a very definite 'Yes'. This time I supported her arm well away from the paper so that she would have to move away from my hand altogether to reach the right circle.

I asked her, 'What are you going to drink now?'

She answered 'Tea', as before.

'What did you drink yesterday?'

'Coffee'.

The pointing was very definite, and was accompanied by a 'so there' glare at the sceptic.

On Friday evening I did my usual end-of-the-week rounds, wandering from ward to ward saying goodnight to all the children, turning on a radio here, handing over a toy there, and I got Annie ready to come home for the weekend. She had had her hospital dinner but when we got home I asked her if she wanted an egg flip, something that she had enjoyed during her last visit. She indicated 'Yes', and while the milk was heating I asked her to show me the circle she would have to point to on the drinks set if she wanted an egg flip. She pointed clearly to the empty circle. As she had stayed up half the night on the last visit I took the precaution this time of reading her *Bedtime for Frances*, a delightful story about a badger with a hundred excuses for not going to bed. She enjoyed it; it is a wonderful story, but I do not think I would have read it to Annie if I had not still been thinking of her as a very young child.

This had been my most exciting week as a teacher. I had come home every night full of the new day's stories: Chris was scarcely able to wait for Annie to come home at the weekend so that he would be able to see for himself what was happening. But even though Annie was doing so well and learning so quickly I was still not crediting her with anything like normal intelligence.

The drinks set was used constantly that weekend, but otherwise we simply spent time showing Annie life in the suburbs. An ordinary person would not have thought that it had a great amount of incident, but it was all extraordinary for Annie. She went to the laundromat, the children's playground, the shops, and the library to see us change our books. It is easy to forget in talking about the institutional environment that it is not just the special events – going to plays and parties – that the children miss out on, it is also the ordinary things like watching a road being dug up or seeing trucks loaded and unloaded, all the experiences that do so much to form our vocabularies. It is a mistake to think that institutionalized children can be de-institutionalized by going on outings to the beach or the theatre. These activities are not as important as all the things we take for granted. When she was at home with me Annie watched me cook. The concepts and vocabulary of cooking are basic to our lives, but in most institutions the children will never see a meal being prepared. It is one of the paradoxes of institutional life that residents may see ballet dancers more often than they see a cook.

Annie had two kinds of education to catch up on: if her academic skills were going to be taken beyond the kindergarten level, her experience of life had to be broadened as well.

ANNIE: When Rosie said she could teach me to talk I knew words would not be enough for what I wanted. Spelling was what I wanted. How to tell Rosie was my problem. Although I was pleased, a quick method of communication was not what I needed. I needed a way of telling people that I knew more than they thought I knew.

CHAPTER SIX

We took Annie back to St Nicholas on Sunday evening and went on to dinner with a friend who is renowned for his ability to provide practical solutions to mechanical problems. I wanted to talk to him about ways to improve Annie's methods of communication and about the possibility of developing a technology that would allow her to be independent. I knew almost nothing about the area. I had talked to people using alphabet boards and word boards - some of the adults I had known at the Spastic Centre sheltered workshop used them - but I had never taught anyone who was using one. I knew nobody who worked with or used advanced technology, and the most sophisticated communications aid I had seen used was a jointed wooden board which could be hung from the back of a wheelchair by a leather handle and which had on it the letters of the alphabet and a few useful words.

What emerged from the evening's discussion had nothing to do with technology. Sean asked me how Annie was remembering her circles. Was it by position, or colour, or the words written on them? I said that I really did not know. There was an obvious and vital question involved. Could Annie recognize words?

The next morning I brought Annie to the playroom for a very important session. When I had written the words on the circles I had done it to remind myself. But I had also hoped that Anne would eventually learn to recognize the words and associate them with the objects and activities they stood for. I was wondering now whether she had done it already.

I told Annie what I was doing and why: I wanted to see if she could recognize words because I wanted to know if she could learn to read. She gave me an enormous smile, but she really did not seem to be very well. I brought in a set of wooden blocks and made cards for 'coffee', 'tea' and 'cordial'. The words were written in black on white in identical printing. I told Annie what was on each card, and I stuck the cards to the blocks and asked her to point to tell me what she had been given to drink earlier in the morning. She pointed correctly to 'coffee'. I shuffled the blocks around. Using blocks meant that her hand could not slide across the words as it could when the words were written on a sheet of paper.

I continued to ask Annie to point to a word that I named from the three written down in front of her. She did this for a while, getting them all right, but she soon lost her enthusiasm and stopped responding. I thought that I was asking too much and that it was possible that she was not sure of her responses when I shuffled the blocks. On the off chance that she was bored, I said, 'We have just been using words. "Coffee" and "tea" and "cordial" are just single words, but when I speak I don't say single words, I say sentences. A sentence is a group of words that go together. "Annie likes coffee" is a sentence: would you like to make a sentence?' She gave me a clear 'yes' response.

I made up blocks with 'Annie' and 'likes' on them, added 'coffee' and put the three blocks together in order: 'Annie likes coffee', telling her what they said. Then I mixed up the blocks and asked her to re-make the sentence. She pointed to the words in the correct order. I went and got an empty scrapbook – a child's book with a picture of a doll on the front. I wrote the sentence in the book, drawing a cup and saucer under it, and with my help Annie coloured it in. I told her she could make another sentence.

'Which words would you like to use?', I asked. 'Do you like tea?'

'Yes', she responded.

'Do you like cordial?'

'No.'

'Well, make up a sentence about tea, then', I suggested.

I put out the four blocks, 'tea', 'Annie', 'coffee', 'likes', and I asked her to point out a new sentence for me. She pointed to 'Annie likes tea.' I copied that into the scrapbook, drew a picture of a teapot, and we coloured it in. Each time I copied a sentence in I put a full stop at the end, explaining this to Annie.

There was something else, I said, that I knew Annie liked, and if she made up a sentence for me she could have one. I wrote 'walk' on a block, and then showed her that I was adding an 's' – we did not say 'Annie likes walk', we said, 'Annie likes walks.' I put out all the blocks and she pointed to 'Annie likes walks' in the correct order. I copied the sentence into the scrapbook without putting a full stop at the end and asked her if there was anything missing. She pointed to the end of the sentence. We drew a street of houses and coloured the houses in. Annie chose 'playground' from the destination set and we went off to the playground, after which it was 11.30 and lunch time.

In the afternoon she developed a temperature which turned into a raging cold, and she was out of commission and very miserable until the following Thursday.

This session was a milestone in my education as much as in Annie's. Clearly my circles were not going to be sufficient for her needs and now that Annie was able to recognize words, it might even be possible for her to learn to read.

And I learned something else that day: there are always

at least two reasons why a student may be unwilling to cooperate, apart from sheer bloody-mindedness. The most obvious is that we are going too fast and asking too much, and the student can't keep up. The other is that we are not going fast enough, and the student is bored. Looking back, I could see that Annie's lack of interest before we started on sentences had something to do with her approaching illness. But it was obvious from the way her performance improved and her enthusiasm returned when I brought up grammar and sentence construction that what I had been asking her to do had bored her.

If Annie could use the circles, I wondered if some of the other children could also learn to use them. While Annie was ill I took the opportunity to try to teach another child to communicate this way. Mark was seventeen and I had always thought that he was the most intelligent of the Beanbaggers. I went through the steps with him in exactly the same way I had with Annie, but he had an advantage over her because he was able to point without having his arm supported. This was very important for my self-confidence. The doubts I had about whether I was influencing Annie's movements subconsciously were irrelevant where Mark was concerned.

Mark learnt the system just as quickly as Annie had, and I started wondering just how many of the very physically handicapped children in St Nicholas could learn to communicate if they were given the chance. The rest of the Beanbaggers were obviously prime candidates for this kind of training, but there were also a number of other children in the hospital who had been left out of the group because of their age (all the Beanbaggers at this time were over the age of ten), but who seemed to me to have a similar level of comprehension.

While Annie was sick I visited her and read her bedtime stories: *Milton the Early Riser* and *Rickie's Birthday*, both for the under-fives. There is no doubt which of us was the slow learner. By Thursday she was well enough to come to the playroom again. I explained that if I were asking for coffee I would probably say, 'I want coffee, please', certainly not just 'coffee'. I explained the pronoun 'I' although her verbal comprehension was so good I assumed she would understand the word despite her inability to use it. I made blocks for 'I', 'want', and 'please', telling Annie what was on them. I mixed up the blocks with the 'coffee' block, and she pointed to 'I want coffee, please.' I copied the sentence into her book and made her some coffee.

When she had finished, I asked her what had happened recently that had interested her. I said I thought it was interesting that she had been sick. I made blocks for 'was', 'sick' and 'yesterday', showing them to her and telling her what was on them, and a block for 'and'. I explained that with 'and' you could say 'I like tea and coffee' without having to say two sentences. From her smile I could see that she thought that was a great idea. I added these four blocks and from her eight blocks she pointed out 'I was sick yesterday.' I copied the sentence into the book with a drawing of her in her cot. I realized then that she did not have a word for me, and I made her a block labelled 'Rosie', telling her she could use it to ask me something. I told her I was sure there was something else she wanted, and if she made a sentence to ask me for it she could have it. I put out six blocks without identifying them: 'Rosie', 'walks', 'I', 'tea', 'want', 'please'. We had not used 'walks' or 'tea' that day. Annie pointed to 'Rosie', which surprised me, and then 'I want walks, please'. When that had been copied into her scrapbook, Annie chose to go to the shops. So off we went, buying some second-hand jeans for Annie to wear next time she came home with us.

Next morning, Friday 6 May, the teachers from Monnington were visiting again. One of them made a videotape of

Anne using the blocks; she loved being taped and enjoyed the replay. She was not told what was on any of the blocks before the session, but she performed perfectly. She remembered all the words she had been given without having to be reminded and made two sentences.

On Monday 9 May I put out all thirteen blocks and asked her what she wanted to drink. She pointed to, 'I want coffee, please.' Again I had not reminded her what was on the blocks. I gave her nine new words: 'am', 'not', 'had', 'Chris', 'a', 'Rosie's house', 'nurse', 'hates' and 'book', in the same way as before. I put all the words on the table in front of Annie and asked her to make some sentences for me. She made four. They were the first sentences she had made without suggestions from me about subjects. She used eight of her nine new words, all of them correctly.

The most interesting of the new sentences was probably 'Annie not Rosie's house yesterday', which was as close to correct as she could manage considering that her grammatical structure was dictated by the words I had chosen. Even with her small number of words she was able to get some subtle meanings across. Her last sentence that morning was 'I want a book, please.' It showed that she was prepared to make the extra effort to include the 'a' and produce an absolutely correct sentence.

The next day Annie chose her drink by picking 'I want tea, please' from the twenty-two words in front of her. Once again, she was not given any reminders and the words were arranged differently from the previous day. She had to remember the word or the shape of the word, not a specific position on the table. After she had drunk her tea I gave her seven new words: 'television', 'at', 'go', 'don't', 'be', 'to', 'shops', mixed them up with her old words and asked her to make a sentence. She was very garrulous, as it happened; she made half a dozen sentences, all of them free and spontaneous, and they made perfectly good sense. One sentence was, 'Annie likes Rosie's house.' Taken with the remark of the day before, I thought she was hinting at something.

By Wednesday Annie was able to use twenty-nine words. She had had five sentence-making lessons, about seven hours of teaching time in all, including the time taken to give her drinks, go to the shops, and make a videotape.

She was doing so well that I decided to check whether she had a concept of words being made up out of building-blocks, that is, out of letters.

I introduced letters in much the same way as I had introduced words. We already had a magnetic board, and at the weekend I had bought a set of children's magnetic letters to go with it. I explained that sentences consisted of words, and that words consisted of letters. With words provided by me she could communicate independently only to a limited extent, because she could only ever use those words I gave her: if she learned to make up her own words out of letters, she could say anything she liked.

'Do you want to learn to spell?', I asked.

She gave me a definite, 'Yes.'

I showed her the letters for Annie, explaining that the 'a' in the set we had was a lower-case one even though the letter at the beginning of a name was usually written with an upper-case one. I made the word 'annie' for her, and then jumbled up the letters and asked her to spell the word by pointing to the letters in the correct order. She could not move the letters around on the board to form a word; she had to point to them in the same way that she had with the word blocks.

As she pointed to each letter I moved that letter to the top of the board, so that a word gradually built up. She spelt 'annie' correctly. I showed her 'rosie', jumbled it up, and asked her to re-make it, which she did with great self-assurance. We then went back to the blocks, and I gave her the day's new words: 'park', 'saw', 'playground', 'drink', 'tired', 'bed', 'today', 'tell', this time spelling them out for her on the board as well as writing them on the blocks. She made a number of sentences and, in a new development, did not want to stop making sentences in order to have a story.

Three sentences were particularly noteworthy in the circumstances: 'I hate Chris yesterday' (in one of the previous day's sentences she had asked him to come to St Nicholas, and he had not been able to make it). I checked it with her yes/no responses, and she had been angry with him for not coming. 'I am Annie' (using the word block to regain her capital letter) and, her last sentence for the day, 'Don't tell Chris please', indicating a certain amount of social awareness. Philip Graves, a handsome young doctor completing his training as a paediatrician with a placement at St Nicholas, was at this session, and Annie's enthusiasm for sentences was possibly motivated by a desire to impress him. There was no doubt that she succeeded.

Now I knew that Annie understood that words were composed of letters, which meant that she should be able to learn to spell. I already knew that she had an excellent visual memory – the way in which she was able to remember the words on the blocks, occasionally using a word for the first time days after it had been introduced, showed that.

On Thursday the sister in charge of Annie's ward came up to see what was going on. I was called away to the telephone, which gave me an excuse to get Annie to work with someone else. I asked the nurse if she would like to work with Annie. When I got back she and Annie had made a sentence, but it was rather peculiar: 'Nurse show bed Rosie's house.' I presumed Annie was saying that she wanted to show the sister where she had slept at my place. 'No', Annie said. The sentence was wrong. We tried again, and this time Annie pointed to 'Annie' instead of nurse and 'likes' instead of 'show', which eventually gave 'Annie likes bed Rosie's house.'

After that I worked with Annie on the full alphabet. I based everything around the *Sesame Street* song, which we played frequently on our cassette. I sang the song as far as each letter, picked the letter out of the jumble in front of us, showed it to Annie, showed her where it came in the words she knew, and stuck it up on the board, ending up with the alphabet in order. I tried asking her a few questions about the letters, but her responses were either wrong or unclear, and I concluded that she did not yet know the alphabet. All Thursday I sang the alphabet song to Annie whenever I could: in the lift, in the bathroom, whenever there was a gap in the conversation. The day's new words on blocks, again spelt out to her on the board, were 'show', 'me', 'you', 'ward', 'my', 'clothes', 'come', and 'the'. We had stopped drawing pictures to go with the sentences in the scrapbook after the first few days. There was not enough space.

On Friday I asked Annie to point to various letters of the alphabet on her board, and she was able to do so correctly. She pointed to 'r' and 'y' quickly when asked, to 'g' after I had sung the song as far as 'g', and to 'n' after quite a pause, as if she was running through the song herself. I did not give her any new words.

On Friday I told the Psychiatrist-Superintendent of St Nicholas, Dr Dennis Maginn, about the work I had been doing with Annie. Dr Maginn was in his late fifties, a large bulky man, with a heavily lined and jowled face. He had been Superintendent since the hospital opened in 1964, and he had given me a great deal of support in 1974. I was nervous when I went to see him because Annie had moved very fast in the last few days, and I was going to tell him about a substantial improvement in a person in whom no improvement had been anticipated.

I knocked at his door and entered without going through his secretary's office. This was the last time I was able to see him so informally. Dr Philip Graves, who had seen Annie on Wednesday, had been to see him on Thursday, and the Superintendent had already heard about her. His first reaction was that I had been trying to keep something from him. But that was only a peripheral issue.

I began to explain what Annie was doing. I was very excited, but he seemed unmoved. I said that although Annie was doing little at this stage her speed at learning compared well with that of the normal children I was teaching as part of the practical work for my Diploma of Education. The word 'normal' broke the Superintendent's composure. He said that if I ever suggested again that any child of normal abilities was living in St Nicholas he would take action against me under the Public Service Act. He said he remembered Anne McDonald from the day of her admission and that what I was suggesting was just not true. He said I was not to mention the work I was doing with Anne to anyone. I asked him to come and see her for himself. He refused.

This was my introduction to an attitude that still persists in the mental health system.

ANNIE: The main reason I used the circles was to make my IQ clear – they gave me very little that was not available from using 'Yes' and 'No'. I would have been upset if Rosie had not moved on to words quickly. The word blocks at least gave me a chance to show that I knew how to make a sentence. With the blocks I could say original things even though their scope was limited by the words I was given.

Chapter Seven

When I began to work with Annie, I was uncertain about what we would be able to achieve. Now I was convinced that Annie could become fully literate, and I began to think about how I could teach her.

One principle seemed to me to be basic. I had learnt it from reading Sylvia Ashton-Warner's splendid book *Teacher*. Working with Maori children in New Zealand, she had discovered that people learn most quickly when they are learning what they really want to know. I tried to use the principle with Annie, to choose words for her that would be as highly motivating as possible: words that would allow her to communicate immediately about the things she was most interested in and give her some control over her environment. Sylvia Ashton-Warner's basic rules apply in any sort of teaching: a child's first reading words must have an intense meaning; a child's first reading books must be made of the stuff of the child's own life. It was for this reason that I kept a book with all the sentences Anne had made. We did not just write the sentences down and forget about them; we read through the book regularly, looking back over what she had done.

Ashton-Warner had also made me aware of the risk of restricting a child to the 'nice' things of life. As well as giving Anne 'like' I also gave her 'hate' very early on. It is important for anyone working with children who cannot speak and who are going to have to use a vocabulary of words, signs or pictures given to them by others to make sure that the children have the means of expressing their dislikes and their frustrations. A basic mistake is to assume that the child has only nice feelings or happiness to express. A handicapped child is more likely to have reason to be frustrated and depressed than an unhandicapped one.

Ashton-Warner's methods had to be modified. She got her pupils to ask her to spell words that they wanted to know, and she discovered that if a child really wanted to know a word, no matter how long or complex it was, it immediately became part of the child's reading vocabulary. It would be a word that the child recognized instantly, what Ashton-Warner called a 'one-look' word.

Annie could not ask for words herself, and I had to guess the words she might respond to. Because she could not talk, I had to use the word blocks to check whether she understood syntax, and so I gave her a number of words that would not usually be among the first learnt by a primary school child learning to read.

I decided that I would try to avoid short-cuts. The temptation in teaching handicapped people is to go for abbreviations, or phonetic spelling, anything to shorten the time taken for communication or lessen the effort. I thought that the initial gains from such short-cuts would have to be paid for dearly later on. I thought if a child got used to an abbreviated structure – if misspellings and abbreviations were accepted regularly from the beginning without checking whether the child could spell – then problems would occur with reading. Phonetic spelling is only acceptable if you are never going to read anything that is not written that way. The other compelling reason for insisting on formal grammatical structure is that because we formulate ideas and communicate them in words, the more sophisticated the grammatical structure at our command, the more sophisticated our means of ordering our thoughts.

Another reason for wanting communication to be in standard English is that it is more socially acceptable. Anne was sixteen when she started to communicate. Most children start a lot earlier. It is cute when a child spells out 'want book' rather than 'I want a book, please.' It is shorter and quicker. But when an adult spells 'want book' an outsider will think he or she is stupid or illiterate. There is so little that Annie can be judged on that she is going to be judged harshly if she makes a mistake.

In thinking about teaching methods I was drawn to a system called *Breakthrough to Literacy*, which works on word recognition in much the same way as Sylvia Ashton-Warner's scheme. *Breakthrough to Literacy* uses a set of word cards which you arrange in order to form sentences. It gives children the joy of making sentences very early on, and it seemed to me that the logical method of teaching Annie to read was by word recognition.

Breakthrough to Literacy was one reading scheme that ignored phonetics, the c-a-t spells cat system, and that appealed to me. Phonetics would be helpful if English was a phonetic language, but it is not: 'kuh, a, tuh' sounds vaguely like 'cat', 'whu, hu, eh, ruh, eh' does not sound like 'where'. I find phonetics ridiculous with normal children; how much more ridiculous they are with children who cannot speak. Nearly all reading schemes use lower-case letters, and I had decided to use them because the differences in shape are greater. On the word cards I had used capitals where they were appropriate: 'Annie', 'I', 'Rosie', and when I wrote Annie's sentences in her book I always gave the first word a capital, explaining why. By Monday 16 May, twenty days after our first session, I was clearer in my mind about how I wanted to teach Annie. I had no idea, however, how soon the next step would come.

The first thing I did at Monday afternoon's session was to ask Annie to point to five letters – 'd', 'j', 'l', 'o', and 'y' – on the magnetic board. She did that with no hesitation. After she had asked for and drunk a cup of tea, I gave her a comprehension test to see if she could recognize the words when I wrote them down in a similar script but a different format. I wrote 'Chris had tea yesterday' in her scrapbook and asked, 'Who had tea yesterday?' and 'When did Chris have tea?' She had to point to the words on the blocks that answered the questions.

She was playing the fool and only pointed to the right answers after a lot of giggling and hand-waving. I wrote a second sentence in her scrapbook: 'Rosie hates television', and asked her, 'What do I hate?' She was still fooling about when Philip Graves came in. When she saw him, she answered the question immediately, full of virtue. I wrote another sentence in the scrapbook to show him what we were doing: 'Annie likes shops.' I asked her, 'What does the sentence say you like?' She pointed immediately to 'shops'.

I did not give her any new word blocks at this session; she had forty-six in front of her every time she made a sentence, and that was about all she could reach. Besides, I wanted to emphasize the importance of learning to spell by showing her how limited her communication was going to be without the ability to spell.

Next day Annie and I had an evening session. She had eaten her dinner and was in her nightdress when I collected her from her cot at about 5.30 and took her to the playroom. I got out the blocks and asked her if she wanted to say anything to begin the session, and she made, 'I hate the ward.' We talked about it, and I suggested various possible meanings, such as, 'I don't like living in a ward' and 'I'm bored

73

in a ward.' I told her that she would not have to stay in St Nicholas for ever and that as soon as she was able to show that she was bright there would be other places for her to go. I told her about the Spastic Centre hostel and Marathon, a school for physically handicapped children. I asked her if she would like to leave St Nicholas and she said, 'No.' I thought that over and told her that I would still visit her and she could still come home with us. I left it at that.

After coffee I told Annie how she could make a lot of new words by changing one letter. I used the word 'at', which she already had on her blocks, and made 'cat', 'fat', 'hat', and 'bat'. I talked about adding an 'e' to the end of '-at' words to make '-ate' words like 'hate' and 'fate'. I thought I might be asking too much, but I wanted her to feel challenged. I asked Annie if she could spell 'I hate fat cats.' I did not show it to her as a sentence, although I had shown her the words before. She hit 'i' and 'h' and looked at me. I asked her for the next letter, and she pointed not to 'a' but to 'f'.

'"F" and what comes after "f"?'

She pointed to 'c', so she had 'i', 'h', 'f', 'c' – initial letters only.

I told her that she had to spell the whole word.

She looked sour but pointed to 'a', 't', 'e' and 'f', 'a', 't'. She started to laugh hysterically and went on laughing while she pointed to 'r', 'o', 's', 'i', 'e', making in all 'I hate fat Rosie.' That is the first sentence Annie ever spelt.

Annie has had a lot of pleasure from that sentence, because I have to say it to people when they ask 'And what was her first sentence?'

We continued our session and talked about '-ck' words like 'lack', 'peck', 'pick' and 'duck'. I was so tired that I could not think of a sentence for Annie to make. I kept asking her to think of one, and she kept saying, 'No.' Eventually I thought of something dull about ducks, and I asked Annie to spell it. She spelt instead 'Rosie is tired.' I had not shown her the word 'is', but she had realized that 'i' is used differently in words like 'bite' and 'bit'. Her use of 'is', a small word and an obvious one, meant that she had broken the code.

Annie had freed herself.

ANNIE: Usually I hated going back to the ward after a session with Rosie, but that night was different. Until that evening I had neither hope nor voice. Now I had both, and I used the night to plan my future. I would be sent to school. My parents would talk to me as a person. I stopped short of imagining leaving St Nicholas. That was too much like heaven to be probable.

I was amazed how quickly spelling followed once I started using circles. Rosie was very perceptive. When she saw me use the circles so well, she hurried me on to words, but she could have stopped there. Mixing the word blocks up each session surprised me. Surely anyone working with a supposedly moderately retarded child would leave the positions constant?

The fact that the blocks were moved gave me a chance to show that I could sight-read words after seeing them once. That stopped us getting stuck on words. Given my word skills, it was obvious to test my ability to use letters; what was amazing was that I was given a chance to show those skills. Rosie allowed structures to develop as they were needed; she never imposed them on me.

Spelling seemed to me the only way dialogue between the handicapped and the vocal could take place. Using any other form of communication lessened my ability to make my own statements. You judge a person by what they say. To be restricted to words chosen by others removes the one means of expressing individuality left to the severely handicapped.

I often thought about ways of communicating while I was incommunicado. Using letters had always seemed better than using symbols or words. When Rosie said she thought she could teach me pictures or symbols, I was worried that that would be all she would try. I worked so hard because that was my only way of showing her that I was brighter than she thought. I am lucky, I have a good visual memory, so I could learn words quickly.

Unless someone makes a jump by going outside the handicapped person's previous stage of communication, there is no way the speechless person can do so. Failure is no crime. Failure to give someone the benefit of the doubt is.

CHAPTER EIGHT

The next day I brought Annie to the playroom at 5 p.m. Philip Graves came with us, the hospital physiotherapist came in, and she and Philip joined Annie and me for coffee. We talked while I gave Annie her coffee, and they stayed for half an hour. When they had gone I asked Annie if she would like to spell something. She responded 'Yes' and pointed to 'I bord.'

'You were bored?,' I asked.

Enthusiastic, 'Yes.'

I showed her 'was' and 'bored' and talked about words ending in '-ed', using words such as 'want' from her blocks. This was the best way for her to learn, I told her. She should try to spell anything she wanted to say, and I would guess what it was and show her how to spell it correctly.

As the point of her using the alphabet board was that she could say whatever she wanted, she could not wait until she learned to spell before she used it. But I was not going to let any incorrect spellings go unchallenged. There was obviously no question of blame if Annie made a mistake, and I made that clear to her, but I wanted her to learn the conventional spelling of a word so that she could use the correct form next time.

A lot of teachers say that to correct children's spelling stifles their creativity. To my mind, not to know how words are spelt or the correct way to construct a sentence will restrict creativity in the long run. For handicapped children who cannot speak, spelling is power, and it is important that they spell correctly so that interpretation by others is easier. It speeds up communication later if you are able to guess the word a child is trying to spell after he or she has hit the first few letters, but you can only do this if you know that the child can spell.

With a licence to go, Annie started to point out a sentence which threw me completely. The first letter of the sentence was 'n' and the next letters were 's', 'd', 'l', 'l', and 'y'. I checked each letter with Annie's yes/no responses, but I could not work out what they meant. I let her go on to the end of this improbable sentence and we ended up with 'Nsdllygoskoolme'. It was the kind of sentence that is easiest to decipher backwards. 'Me', that was a word; 'skool', a classic misspelling; 'go', that made sense; 'something go skool me'. 'Sally!' The 'd' had been pointed to in mistake for the 'a'. 'Sally go school me.' 'N?' 'When!' I had asked Annie to spell words as they sounded, using bits of phonetics from words she knew. How do you symbolize the 'wh' in 'when' unless you know how it is spelt? There is no letter that sounds like 'wh'. The only letter that comes out solidly is the 'n', showing again the disadvantage of phonetic spelling.

I asked Annie if she meant 'when', and she indicated 'Yes.' I showed her how to spell it properly. Translated and expanded, the sentence read, 'When will Sally go to school with me?' Sally was our neighbour's little girl, in her first year at primary school, and she was just learning to read and write. Annie obviously thought that they could start having lessons together. The next sentence she spelt perfectly: 'You tell Sally when.' I was to make a date with Sally for a joint session. Annie still wanted to say more, despite my pleas for mercy, and very quickly (for Annie, it took about ten minutes) pointed out, 'You tell me what she ses.'

It was interesting that 'what' was spelt correctly, presumably by extrapolation from 'when' and 'was'. Annie's memory and generalizing ability were very good.

I had been pleading for mercy because of my back. Supporting Annie in the baby buggy for any length of time was the most excruciating procedure. Her head exerted enormous backwards extension pressure on my left arm, which really worked for its living, and I had to bend over at an awkward angle to support her right arm at the appropriate height; she was using a kindergarten-height table. I had to do this for up to half an hour a sentence, depending on how tense she was, how quickly she was able to move, and how long the sentence was. I could never understand why the people who thought I was making the whole thing up did not ask themselves why I had not chosen a more comfortable method.

I was hoping that Annie would pick up some spelling by reading simple books with me, and I tried to select books that seemed interesting and appropriate. Annie certainly did not fit the profile of a normal middle-class five-year-old living at home, and it would have been silly to treat her as if she did.

On Thursday we looked through *Where Is Wiffen?* from the Bowmar series for new readers. Annie was taken with Jimmy, the hero. I showed her the picture, said a bit about it and then asked, 'What do the words say?' I read the words slowly, pointing to each one with Annie's finger and checking to see that she was watching. Occasionally I commented on a word, but only after reading all the other words on a page and not at enough length to disrupt the story. I chose *Where is Wiffen?* because it is about a dog, and the children at the hospital had just seen some puppies.

When we had finished the book I asked Annie if she would like to make a sentence about a puppy. She ignored the question and spelt out 'Feed me, Rosie.' Her request alarmed me, and we stopped and discussed it. I knew about some of the feeding problems Annie was having; after all, one of the reasons I had taken her home in the first place had been that she had been losing weight. But it seemed to me impossible to justify feeding her myself. It would have been arrant favouritism, and I did not have the time. I was responsible for the administration of playgroups for about ninety children in St Nicholas; I was working with a number of children myself each week, about thirty multiply handicapped children in addition to Annie; and I was trying to do my part-time course for the Diploma of Education. There were not enough hours in the day to fit in everything that needed to be done.

I told Annie that I would feed her if I had time, but I could only feed her three lunches and one dinner a week at the most, and I probably would not be free for those four meals a week on a regular basis.

For Annie's first few spelling sessions I had used the spelling board on an easel at an angle to the table. This time I decided to see how she went using it flat, and that was the way she had spelt the last sentence. Now she spelt, 'Ce I can do it.' I showed her 'see' and talked about it. I asked her if she liked the board down, and she said 'Yes.' But she also said she liked it up. I told her to choose between up and down. She spelt 'doun'. We talked about 'down', and how it was different from 'out'; then very stupidly, I took the 'd' off 'down' and made 'own', which sounds nothing like it. I put off teaching frown, moan, thrown, stone, shown, and alone for another day.

On Friday I decided that as Annie and Mark and his friend Angela, who was also able to point clearly without any arm support, were doing so well (Mark was also making sentences from words), I would introduce the circles to the other six Beanbaggers. They all performed well, and they all chose drinks using a set of circles.

Annie and I had a very trying session in the evening,

because I could not make head or tail of what she was saying. We had not got all the bugs out of the system, by any means.

On Tuesday 24 May I picked up Annie straight after dinner, at about 4.30. She was crying, and when I took her to the playroom she pointed out, 'I hanik gec any pooding' which translated without much difficulty into, 'I didn't get any pudding' and was a lament from the heart. I was not sure if it was strictly true, but I stewed up some apples for her anyway. While they were stewing I told Annie about '-it' words, '-ite' words and '-ight' words. I asked her if there was anything else she wanted to say, and she went on to spell 'I can't feed myself', which obviously referred to her earlier request that I feed her. She was still very thin, and weighed little more than 12 kilograms.

Not long afterwards, I did start to feed Annie. A nurse who had been having psychiatric problems was rostered to feed her, and she mistreated her very badly. Annie spelt out to me that the nurse had slapped her, and I reported it to the Director of Nursing: the first patient complaint, I would think, in the history of St Nicholas Hospital. The Director said he had already received a report from the sister in charge of the ward. The sister told me that Annie had almost suffocated as the food was spooned in. She had finished up with food all over her, and she had been terribly upset. The incident jarred my conscience and I began to feed Annie regularly.

The nurse stopped looking after Annie for the next few weeks, but after that she seemed to be in charge of Annie at all times. When Annie was moved to another ward, the nurse went with her. The nurse later went on night duty in Annie's ward, which meant there was even less chance to keep an eye on her. Annie could not run away, could not retaliate, and could not complain freely. When Annie told me she was scared, I raised the matter with a senior member of the nursing staff. I was told that the nurse was being put in charge of Annie deliberately to see if she would do it again, so that they would have grounds for sacking her.

On Tuesday I also brought Mark to the playroom. He had been using a word board very well, and I wanted to see if he could learn to spell. Annie found it very amusing to watch someone go through all the processes she had outgrown so recently.

The next day we had a dance troupe performing at the hospital, and Annie enjoyed it enormously. She was not able to sit in the pusher for any length of time, and I held her on my lap in a flexed position so she could see: it was an exhausting business, because the constant pressure of her muscular spasm pushed her out into a bow against my restraining arms.

On the Friday morning, 27 May, Annie came to the playroom for a quick session to bring the videotape up to date. She was very glad of the chance to show off her new-found spelling skills to the teachers from Monnington who had met her for the first time only a month before.

I had arranged to have Annie for the weekend. I collected her from the ward in the afternoon and we went off to catch the train to a small town in south-western Victoria called Birregurra where I have a cottage. The train took two hours to travel the 130 kilometres from Melbourne, but Annie enjoyed it. On Saturday morning we went for a walk around the town. Birregurra is one of those country towns with a very wide main street and almost no traffic; Annie was most impressed. We saw cows, horses, kittens, and sheep, and Anubis, the dog, went for a swim in the river.

In the afternoon we went to visit some of my relatives. They were excruciatingly tactless about Annie, in her hearing, despite my having told them repeatedly and explicitly that she could understand everything they said.

'Well, if it was a puppy you'd knock it on the head, wouldn't you?', one of them said.

Another was not only tactless but senile and deaf and kept repeating loudly like a cracked record, 'If it was my child I'd kill it and you couldn't blame me.'

Annie bore up well enough at the time. She did not cry or carry on, and I thought that perhaps she had given up worrying about remarks like these.

Back at the cottage she ate a porterhouse steak with mushrooms for dinner, and I started to chat for her benefit about the Australian system of government. When I said that the leader of the party in power in Canberra was called the Prime Minister, Annie started jumping up and down in her pusher.

'Is there anything you want to say?', I asked.

'Yes', she responded.

I looked at her and tried to work out what it could be.

'Oh, you know the name of the Prime Minister?'

'Yes.'

I asked her to spell it. Carefully and with complete assurance she spelt 'Malcolm Fraser.' I gave her no clues. Presumable she had seen Fraser's name spelt out on the television screen. It was the only place she could have learnt the spelling of Malcolm.

I had always told her that after she had learnt to spell I would be able to ask her questions and find out what she knew. That evening, for the first time, we got a taste of her interest in the world outside St Nicholas and of the amount of information she had collected about it.

I went on with my politics lecture. When I got to the Leader of the Opposition Annie jumped up and down again. I offered her the board and she spelt out 'Gough Whitlam' correctly. We moved on from federal politics to state politics, and as soon as I mentioned the Premier the same thing happened. She spelt out 'Hamer.'

'Right, do you know the name of the Leader of the Opposition in Victoria?', I asked.

She spelt 'Cive Holding.' His name was Clyde, but she may not have seen his name on television and only heard it on the radio.

Chris was enormously excited. This was the first time he had really seen Annie spelling out anything more complicated than what she wanted to drink. We were usually so busy at the weekend that we did not have time to use the communications board very often. Now we had broken into a whole new area and discovered something about Annie that we had not known before.

This evening's performance had, once again, completely changed my perception of Annie. Whether or not she was functioning at a level appropriate for her age, her interests were certainly appropriate.

When we were all in bed Annie started to cry unconsolably. I went to her room and tried to comfort her, without success. I tried to find out what was wrong so I could do something about it. It was not any of the obvious things: she was not feeling sick, she did not have a headache, and she did not have a stomach-ache. Finally I had to ask her to try to spell out what it was all about. It was a horrible thing to do. Annie was terribly upset and crying as if her heart would break. But it was the only thing possible. I had to say, 'Right, you're going to have to take fifteen minutes to spell out something that will give me some idea of what's upsetting you, and I can't help you until you do.'

When she was seated at the board, she spelt out 'Fewtur.' 'Future.' She was worried about what would become of her. She had not just skipped over the comments about how she should be killed; she had bottled them up, and they had proved too much for her. Only a few days ago I had been telling her that she would not have to stay in St Nicholas all her life. And here she was outside with people who thought she should be killed. It was no wonder that she was worried about her future. I talked about it at length. It was on this night that I first mentioned to Annie the possibility of writing a book. I told her that she had a lot to offer people who were handicapped like herself, and I thought that one day she and I could write a book about our experiences together. I promised her that Chris and I would see that she did not have to stay in St Nicholas for ever.

We came back to Melbourne on Sunday night and took Annie back to the ward.

We had another videotaping session at St Nicholas on Monday, this time with some of the social workers lending a hand. After Annie had answered a couple of questions, a social worker took over supporting her arm. It was an illustration of how people not used to working with physically handicapped children get so caught up in extraneous details that they miss what is going on. They thought up the questions, so that it could not be said that I had rehearsed Annie in a narrow range of answers. I was to go outside the room and a social worker was to support Annie's arm so she could answer questions put by another social worker, who did not know the answers. From outside the room I could see Annie's back through the glass door. One of the questions was, 'What is the name of Rosie's neighbour's eldest daughter?' Annie tried and tried to reach the 's'. I could see it through the window. It is a difficult letter for her, because it is in the bottom left-hand corner of her board and reaching for it tends to send her arm into cramp. After a while I was called back in again, and the social workers said that they had not been able to get anything.

'What was the name?', one of them asked.

'Sally', I replied.

'She was never over near the "s",' she said, 'at any stage.'

That was not true. I had been able to see it through the window, and I ran back the tape for them. I was able to stop the videotape to get a still picture of Annie's hand resting clearly on the 's'. For some reason, they had quite genuinely thought she had never been near it; perhaps because they had been concentrating on other things – working the camera, holding her arm – they had not noticed.

We tried it again and it failed in the same way. The social workers were upset, but it was not their fault. They had no experience in this area and were only trying to do me a favour.

ANNIE: I was utterly shattered when Rosie's relative said if I was a puppy I would be knocked on the head. Sweeping assessments I was used to, but this was the most hurtful I'd had. I had often wished someone would kill me, but I didn't feel other people should want me dead. What hurt me most was the realization that people outside St Nicholas felt the same about handicapped people as the nurses did.

Since then I have realized that most people do not feel as strongly as Rosie's relative did. They just wish we would keep off the streets. Rosie and her friends are the only people I have met who think that we should be out and about.

Chapter Nine

On Wednesday 1 June Elizabeth, one of the teacher aides, came in while I was working with Annie, and we joked about Annie's knowledge of current affairs. I asked Annie which party she would vote for, Labor or Liberal, warning her that her education could stop right there if she gave the wrong answer. She spelt 'labor'.

When Elizabeth left we went through a Bowmar book called *Do you Suppose Miss Riley Knows?* word by word, and I gave Annie a drink. Then I took all the magnetic letters off the board and told Annie I wanted to see how much she knew about numbers.

That is the way I put it to her as I was chalking numbers on her magnetic board, and the way I put it is probably quite important. I was not going to start to teach her about numbers, I was not going to ask her if she knew anything about numbers, I was going to see *what* she knew about numbers. On the basis of her performance over the past few weeks I thought she would probably know something.

I had taught her basic counting. The Beanbaggers had done activities like pile blocks together, count fingers and toes, and sing the number song from *Sesame Street*. Each child had painted over pictures I had drawn of different numbers of objects. The pictures had the numbers written at the bottom of them to make the purpose clear to any observer, not because I expected the children to recognize the numbers, and I stuck them on the wall of the activity room to go with a number frieze I had bought. I expected Annie to know how to count, and I thought that if she did not recognize the numbers already she would learn to do so quickly.

I had checked the Beanbaggers' counting ability by making two groups of blocks on a tray. I insisted on groups not piles because you have to count groups, but you can get piles by height. I showed the groups to a child, and asked him to point to the group that had five blocks. The child turned his head or eyes or pointed to one lot or another. We had been doing this for a time, and I had been using counting whenever it came up naturally. 'Right, that's one, two, three of you who have asked for coffee; one, two, three, four, five of you who want tea, one, two chocolate milk; that's ten of you altogether,' I would say.

The children did have access to the concept of one number being made up of other variable groups of numbers, which is the basis of addition. Every time I was putting out cups and saucers or dividing up a punnet of strawberries I would count: 'one, two, three ... children and one, two, three ... plates', putting a plate on each child's knee to show the one-to-one correspondence (and to hold the strawberries). 'One for you, and one for you, and one for you, eleven kids with one strawberry each is eleven strawberries doled out.

This was all just part of the running patter that I kept up throughout all the Beanbaggers' sessions. I was conscious that it was important for me to talk to the children as much as possible; it did not really matter whether they understood every word I was saying. I hoped they would understand most of it, and I tried to pitch it at what I thought was an appropriate level. Although I did not expect them to know the numbers up to twenty-two, I did not think it would do them any harm to know that there were numbers as big as that, and that there were numbers beyond the ones they had been taught, even if they did not know precisely what they symbolized. I wanted them to know that when somebody used the word thirty-six, say, that it was a number and referred to a quantity in the same way as ten did. I used to count up to a hundred every now and again just so they could hear the words and understand that there was some sequence involved.

Later on, I was to do this a lot more, in a lot more detail, and with a much more definite aim in view, but this introduction to really basic number concepts was aimed only at increasing their linguistic comprehension.

For Annie I took the magnetic letters off the board and wrote two rows of numbers on it with chalk, thus:

Diagram 7

$$1 \quad 2 \quad 3 \quad 4 \quad 5 \quad 6 \quad 7$$
$$8 \quad 9 \quad 10 \quad 11 \quad 12 \quad 13 \quad 14$$

and I told Annie what they were as I wrote them on. When she had finished her coffee I drew three dots on the board with chalk:

Diagram 8

• • •

and I asked her to count them and point to the number that symbolized them. I helped her by placing her finger on each dot in turn. I was not sure how much she could comprehend just by looking, and I thought that if she could count she would probably need a one-to-one correspondence. Then I supported her arm and she pointed to the answer she wanted to give, which was 3. I added three more dots:

Diagram 9

•   •   •

•   •   •

---

and went through the procedure again. When I asked her to indicate the number that stood for that number of dots, Annie pointed to 6. Unable to resist improving on her performance, I talked about 'three plus three equals six' and 'three multiplied by two equals six'. I had added three dots to three dots and so we now had two lots of three. Then I added two more:

Diagram 10

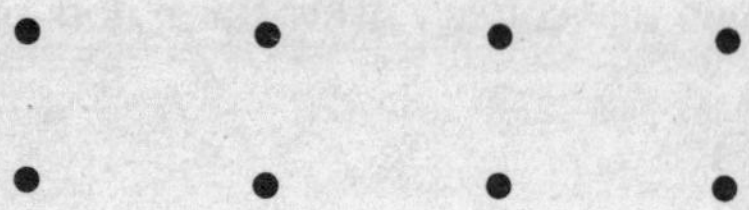

•   •   •   •

•   •   •   •

This time I did not put her fingers on the board. I wanted to see whether she could count the dots without touching them. She pointed to 8. I added five more dots and she pointed to 13. I was pleased because it showed that she could cope with two-digit numbers – positional notation.

I thought I would try Annie on a simple sum. I wrote it out in figures, thinking that I could translate it into dots for her if she could not manage it. The sum was 2 + 3, written in ordinary arithmetic notation. I told her what the symbols plus (+) and equals (=) mean and told her the sum in as many different ways as possible: two and three, two plus three, gives, equals. Annie pointed to 5 with no hesitation.

At this stage I called in Elizabeth, the teacher aide, so that we would have an observer. It was important for two reasons: if Annie was doing this all by herself it was remarkable and somebody else should be there to witness it; and I was worried that Annie was not doing it by herself. Perhaps I *was* moving her arm unintentionally. We went on with the series of sums: 4 + 5 = 9; 7 + 4 = 11. Annie could add up; furthermore, she understood the concept of a carrying figure.

I decided to try Annie on subtraction, which really had not come up in the Beanbaggers' sessions except by implication (if there are ten cups of cordial and I have given out seven, that means there are three to go). I had certainly not given it even the same low-level emphasis that I had given addition. I wrote on the board 10 − 8; Annie pointed to 2.

We went straight on to multiplication: 3 x 4 = 12. And then division: 15 ÷ 3 = 5. Then I gave Annie a more difficult addition: 23 + 4, which involved her in pointing to two figures because 27 was not on the board. She pointed to 2 and then to 7. As I wrote each sum I said it to her in as many forms as I could think of, and I explained each new sign as it came up.

You can see something from the sequence of sums. I asked her to do four lots of counting, three lots of addition, one subtraction, one multiplication, one division and one complex addition. The more Annie did the more obvious it became that it was very easy for her and that we were working in an area in which she was very competent. The look of triumph on her face was enough to convince us that we did not need to examine the more difficult operations in the same detail we had given her counting.

Annie's evident pleasure was a fairly convincing indication that I was not helping her get the answers, but I was still very worried. Only six weeks ago I had thought of Annie as having an IQ of less than 50. Elizabeth was convinced that I had not been moving Annie's arm or suggesting the answers in other ways - moving the board, say - but because of my doubts I suggested that we try a test. I would leave the room, Elizabeth would write a sum on a piece of paper and show it to Annie. When I came back I would hold Annie's arm while she pointed to the answer. But when we attempted the test Annie was restless, mucked about, made what I would usually have regarded as definite pauses over wrong numbers, and finally hit the answer, which was 8. It was not satisfactory. The second question was no better, but for the third she steadied up and pointed to 2 and 3 - the numbers that had been written down - and 5, the answer. I was not entirely happy, because her pointing was not as clear as it might have been, and I got Elizabeth to write down just one number while my back was turned. Annie pointed to this clearly enough. She had been working for more than two hours, and it was nearly lunch time. I thought this might have had something to do with her lowered performance.

After we had taken Annie back to the ward I became very depressed and uncertain about what had happened. Elizabeth was reassuring, but I still found it hard to believe, particularly after her performance at the end.

In retrospect I can see why Annie was unhappy with the tests and played up when we asked her to do them. Having shown that she was able to do things that were completely unexpected of her and that she had taught herself things that normal children do not usually learn without help, she was given no credit for it. I doubted her. The extent of her performance had not increased my faith in her ability, it had diminished it and made me doubt whether she was doing anything at all. I needed reassurance, and the only way I could get it was by admitting to Annie that I doubted her. Annie found it almost unbearable.

In the afternoon, there was a case conference on Mark. A case conference involved a discussion of the child by a representative of every discipline concerned with the child's care: doctor, physiotherapist, social worker, and so on. Case conferences were new to the hospital then and were discontinued later. This conference had been requested by Philip Graves and myself. I showed a short videotape of Mark using a word board. It was not very clear, as I was the first to admit, because I had to be teacher, producer, and camera operator, but it gave some idea of the kind of work we were doing, and the fact that I was out in front holding the camera emphasized Mark's independence. In any case, the tape was received with a complete lack of interest; nobody debated its validity, or its implications. No suggestions were made about changes in Mark's care. As with Annie, none of the people with power in the hospital wanted to come and see Mark working. They made it clear that they did not want to see the children, they wanted videotapes.

The next morning I received a memorandum from the administration asking to see a videotape of Anne at the end of the month, and telling me that the tape was not to be shown to an outsider before then. On the same day I was told that I could not take time off without pay to complete my course for the Diploma of Education. It was suggested that I become a half-time employee or, preferably, resign altogether.

I brought Annie, Mark and Angela to the playroom after tea to try to improvise a sling to support Annie's arm. If she could work with her arm in a sling it would negate suggestions that I was manipulating her answers. Angela and Mark had never needed their arms supported and did not have the same problem. The sling was made from a piece of nylon suspended from a baby's swing frame. I suspect it soon became uncomfortable, and it certainly substantially inhibited Annie's vision. Annie tried it nonetheless, first pointing to letters on request and then completing a number of sums.

Her answers were clear enough, but they were given very slowly: $16 \div 4 = 4$, $4 \times 2 = 8$, $15 + 14 = 29$, $18 \div 3 = 6$, just repeats of yesterday's session.

I decided to take a big leap and move on to fractions. I told Annie what fractions were, and I wrote down a sum: $½ + ½$. I said it in every way I could: two halves, a half plus another half. She pointed clearly to 1, but she was slow. The next few sums took even longer, either because they were harder or because she had been in the sling for an hour and was flagging. I gave her $⅔ + ⅓$ and she pointed to 2. Now $½ + ½$ is easy enough, because you talk about halves in ordinary conversation. I had cut many apples in half for the children's fruit salads and told them what I was doing. The first sum needed nothing more than linguistic knowledge. But the sum, $⅔ + ⅓$, was very different: Annie had to be able to reduce her answer to a whole number. I had to explain the notation; for example, the way you write a half as one divided by two. That would have given any reasonably able child a clue to the answer to the first sum. For $⅔$ I made it clear that you could write more than a whole number in fraction form, which was another clue, but not an explanation.

The question left unanswered was where Annie had learnt all this. I talked to her about it – not on the board, she was tired – through her yes/no responses. When I asked her if she had learnt multiplication and division from *Sesame Street* she gave me a half-yes, half-no answer. When questioned her further, I established that she had learnt the numbers and basic addition from *Sesame Street* but that she had extrapolated multiplication and division from addition and subtraction. That did not explain how she had learnt fractions, which in the St Nicholas environment I found almost beyond belief. Later I decided she had at least got a start from a picture book called *Drei Äpfel* (a story about three apples on a plate), which I had shown the group often. In the story, one of the apples was peeled, one was bitten, and one was cut into quarters. I used to match the apples in the book with real apples on a plate to try to reinforce the connection between real life and pictures and to emphasize the number concepts involved. When cutting the apple into quarters I emphasized that one apple contained two halves and four quarters, two quarters to a half. I did this not because I contemplated the children ever doing mathematics at that level, but because we talk of halves and quarters in everyday life. We talk about 'half a bar of chocolate', 'half time' in football, and we say 'quarter past three'. I wanted the children to have a concept of a half as being a part of something and a quarter as being a smaller part. The apple lesson was part of a general lesson on fruit, and we chopped up all kinds of fruit to make a big bowl of fruit salad. When I thought about Annie and fractions, the lesson on fruit seemed to be the only explanation.

I was both right and wrong. In 1979 Annie spelt out 'Salad was the catalyst. Joey extended it and suggested eighths and sixteenths. He was brighter than me.'

Joey was the boy who had died in 1976, and I was sure, looking back, that he must have been intelligent too. Now Annie had confirmed it. Joey had died without ever communicating with an adult. His 'noises' had apparently made sense to the children.

On Sunday I picked Annie up at the hospital to take her out to lunch with the friends we had visited the first weekend Annie had been home. There were two children at lunch, Damien aged about nine and Bill aged about five. Damien had met Annie on the last visit, and when he had heard that she was coming to lunch he had made her one of those woolly balls you get by winding wool around cardboard doughnuts. I was afraid that she might think it too babyish for her, but she spelt out 'Thank you' happily enough. Damien and Bill thought Annie's board work was fascinating, and they could not wait to see her do more. Damien asked her what she had for breakfast, and despite my telling him he insisted that she spell it herself. When she had gone as far as 'por' he jumped in and said, 'The rest's easy – just "idge",' which gave Annie a chance to give him a scathing look and point decisively to the second 'r' before spelling 'idge'.

Bill set Annie some sums. He had just started numbers at primary school. He gave her three very simple additions, and after I had taken the letters off the board and written up the digits, Annie pointed to the answers immediately. She set Bill some sums, carefully keeping away from the numbers he had used and was very amused when he could not do them.

After lunch we all drove down to the beach and went to the playground nearby before calling at my house for an egg flip on the way back to St Nicholas.

On Monday evening we sorted through the sea-shells we had collected at the beach on Sunday, and then I read Annie a couple of Hilaire Belloc's *Cautionary Tales*, which she enjoyed well enough. At some stage I ducked off to the toilet, which is in hearing distance of the activities room. When I came back I set up the board and asked Annie to spell out as much as possible about yesterday. She spelt instead 'You piss lots' which led us to a discussion of euphemisms. That sentence also resurfaced many times, and I was cross-examined on it in the Supreme Court two years later.

She went on to spell, 'List errors, Rosie', and when I asked her which errors she was referring to she added 'in my writing'. When I asked her why she wanted me to list her errors she spelt 'so we teach others'. I explained that I had been taking notes of what we had done and showed her in her scrapbook the way I had noted down what she had intended to say in textacolour and her mistakes in biro.

Annie made it clear that she wanted to say something else and spelt, 'When will we start the book?' I told her that there were two answers. One was that we had already begun it. What she and I were writing would be part of it. The other was that we needed more advanced technical equipment for her so that she could write without my help, and I mentioned electric typewriters.

I had promised Annie that we would talk about fractions, but we did not have time. I was still working with numbers of other children and was fitting in Annie whenever I could, usually in the evening after the other children were in bed. My working day officially ended at five o'clock, and after that I was free to work with anyone I liked. Annie occasionally went for days without a chance to spell out anything on the alphabet board.

Over the next few months the situation got worse. As I taught more children to spell I had less time to work with any of them individually, which was what they needed if they were going to have an opportunity to use the spelling I had taught them.

On Tuesday 7 June I set Annie her first homework. During the evening I talked to her about fractions, drawing rectangles and dividing them up so she could see the one-quarter equals two-eighths kind of relationship. I explained how we could add fractions with unlike bases using lowest common denominators, and I worked out a sum involving thirds and quarters in front of her in full, working through all the possible denominators from four up. She seemed rather bored, but I felt it was important to make the notion of fractions concrete.

When I took her back to her cot, I set her some homework

using the cot bars. There are eleven bars to a cot side, dividing each side into ten parts, so I asked Annie to think about tenths and their relationships, pointing out only that two-tenths equals one-fifth. Two days later I checked the homework by setting her some sums. I said to her, 'Point to two fractions that mean the same amount.' They were multiple-choice sums, and Annie's responses are circled:

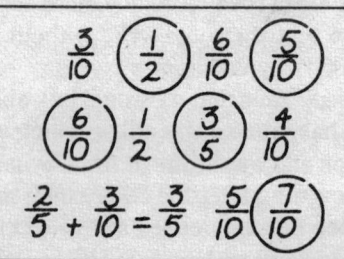

Diagram 11

$$\frac{3}{10} \quad \boxed{\frac{1}{2}} \quad \frac{6}{10} \quad \boxed{\frac{5}{10}}$$

$$\boxed{\frac{6}{10}} \quad \frac{1}{2} \quad \boxed{\frac{3}{5}} \quad \frac{4}{10}$$

$$\frac{2}{5} + \frac{3}{10} = \frac{3}{5} \quad \frac{5}{10} \quad \boxed{\frac{7}{10}}$$

Her responses were clear and definite. For her next batch of homework I drew twelve lines on a piece of paper and stuck it on her cot, asking her to think about twelfths. I pointed out that twelfths were more interesting than tenths because there were more permutations and combinations.

On Thursday 9 June I had a meeting with some of the Education Department staff to discuss whether they had anyone prepared to work with Mark and Angela. I did not have time to give them the attention they needed and both were now spelling using an alphabet board. Because they were both able to point without assistance they were both much more 'saleable' than Annie. No one could suggest that they were being manipulated; furthermore, they were physically easier to work with. And it seemed a good idea to involve other people in the programme so that it could not be said that I was the only person who was able to communicate with the children.

Margaret Tenney had recently started to work at St

Nicholas as head of the education staff, and I arranged for her to come and see Annie.

Margaret asked Annie if she watched television.

Annie replied 'Roots', which was the name of a major series that had just been shown in Australia.

'Roots', I said, 'what roots – tree roots?'

Annie spelt 'TV'.

I asked her to tell us what *Roots* was about.

'Slaves', replied Annie.

'Where did the slaves come from?', I asked. I had not seen the show, but I expected her to answer 'Africa'.

Annie spelt out a long name, which she claimed was the name of the village. Margaret had not seen the show either, and we did not know if she was right.

We discussed the plot, and when I asked Annie the name of the slave ship she pointed to 'l' as the first letter. Then the telephone rang, and we had to end the session.

Next day Margaret came in with an article on *Roots*; the name of the ship was the *Lord Ligonier*, but the name of the village was not mentioned. In front of Annie, Margaret said that she thought Annie's 'l' must have been a coincidence.

This was one of our standard problems: people who doubted the children were always so sure of themselves that they openly expressed their scepticism in front of them. It did not occur to them that if they were wrong they were terribly rude, and that they were making it very difficult for the children to respond to them. How do you talk to someone who tells you that they are convinced that you cannot talk? What are they going to 'hear' when you try to talk? The problem was exacerbated by the children's abnormal muscular tension, a typical feature of cerebral palsy. A person affected by cerebral palsy who is nervous, angry, or upset is likely to have increased muscle spasm, which makes it much more difficult to perform physical tasks.

Annie's muscles tightened automatically when she was working in front of someone she knew did not believe in her. She had a lot more difficulty than usual moving her arm. It tended to cramp more often, and when she pointed she was not very clear. This played into the hands of sceptics and confirmed their disbelief.

There are rooms with one-way windows where children can work without being aware of observers, but we had none at St Nicholas. Even now, psychologists claiming to do an unbiased assessment of these children sit down directly in front of them while they are working and pass comments on them and their performance. Even professionals in the area seem to work on the assumption that if children cannot speak they cannot hear either. An 'expert' recently asked me to ask Leonie something to see how she would react. It would be difficult, I pointed out, to get a natural reaction. Leonie had been present when the expert told me what to ask her. Leonie's difficulty in communicating with people did *not* mean that she had difficulty in hearing them.

After Margaret left I checked Annie's mathematics and gave her some more to do over the weekend. We began work on powers, which I explained were shorthand for a number multiplied by itself. I wrote down this series:

Diagram 12

$$2 \times 1 = 2 = 2^1$$
$$2 \times 2 = 4 = 2^2$$
$$2 \times 2 \times 2 = 8 = 2^3$$
$$2 \times 2 \times 2 \times 2 = 16 = 2^4$$

---

and pointed out that the superscript was the number of twos to the left of the sum. There was a certain irony in putting this kind of thing on the bars of a baby cot in a hospital for the severely retarded.

St Nicholas had advantages in getting homework done; however boring or difficult or uninteresting it may have seemed to an ordinary child, the work was all that Annie had to occupy her from 4.30 each afternoon to 7.30 in the morning. Any homework I have ever set has always been done.

We took Annie out of the hospital on Saturday afternoon and went to the zoo and then back to our house for dinner. Chris had found a long newspaper article on *Roots*, and to keep Annie entertained while I was cooking I propped it up in front of her as she lay on the floor in the dining-room. Annie said she was reading it, and when I tiptoed up to look she certainly seemed to be. When I thought she had finished the article I asked her some comprehension questions.

'Alex Haley wrote one well-known book before *Roots*. He helped a famous black American write his autobiography. What was the name of the man he helped?'

Annie spelt 'Malcolm X'.

'Who were the wise old men who knew the tribe's history and told Alex Haley about his family's background in Africa?'

'Griots', she replied.

These words were in small print in the middle of columns: Malcolm X was mentioned about half way through the piece, and the griots appeared in the last two columns. The word 'griots' had no capital letter and did not stand out at all. Annie had proved that she was able to read an ordinary newspaper article. Now she could be called literate.

It was 13 June 1977, less than a month after Annie had spelt out 'I hate fat Rosie' and about seven weeks after Annie's first visit home. There were undoubtedly many words she had never seen written and would not be able to spell, and there were probably quite a few words whose meaning she was able to guess from their context but whose sound she did not know. She had reached a reading level that would have satisfied most people teaching ordinary sixteen-year-olds.

Annie's mathematical ability continued to astonish me. On Wednesday 15 June I questioned her on powers. I set up the board in this way:

Diagram 13

$$1 \quad 2 \quad 3 \quad 4 \quad 5$$
$$6 \quad 7 \quad 8 \quad 9 \quad 0$$

I wrote the basic ten numbers on the board and it became the standard board which all the children have used since.

I set some questions for Annie, and her answers were all correct. These were the problems and answers:

Diagram 14

$$2^3 = 8$$
$$3^3 = 27$$
$$4^6 \div 4^4 = 16$$

Annie had worked out for herself the principle involved in this sort of division: to divide one number with a superscript by the same number with another superscript, you subtract one superscript from the other. She was able to generalize from what she saw, form a hypothesis, and test it. In this case she hit upon the correct hypothesis.

To check her homework on fractions I set out this problem and put down four answers for her to choose from:

Diagram 15

$$\frac{3}{32} + \frac{1}{8} + \frac{1}{4} = \frac{5}{44} \quad \frac{5}{32} \quad \frac{15}{32} \quad \frac{17}{8}$$

Annie chose: $\frac{15}{32}$

On Monday I talked to Annie about time. I had noticed her looking up at the clocks when I mentioned time: if I said it was lunch time, or half past five, she would look up. I suspected that she had some idea about telling the time but I thought she would be uncertain of the finer points, such as 1.35 being the same as twenty-five to two.

Because I try to ask questions which I think have a good probability of being answered correctly – I want children to experience success, not failure – I talked briefly about time with Annie and gave her a clock face marked in this way before asking her any questions:

Diagram 16

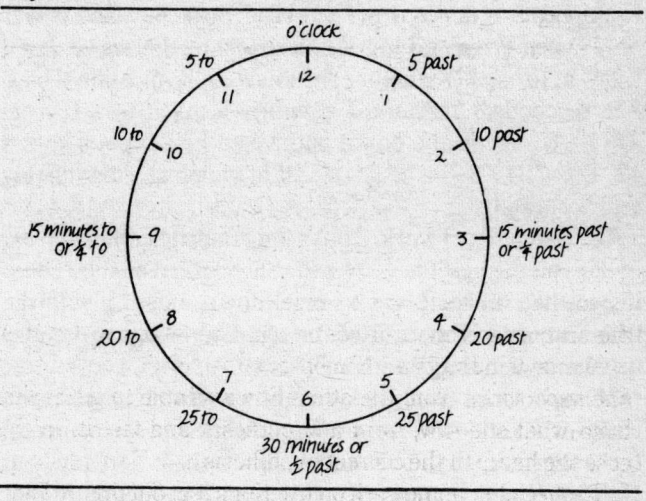

Clock face showing:
- 12: o'clock
- 1: 5 past
- 2: 10 past
- 3: 15 minutes past or ¼ past
- 4: 20 past
- 5: 25 past
- 6: 30 minutes or ½ past
- 7: 25 to
- 8: 20 to
- 9: 15 minutes to or ¼ to
- 10: 10 to
- 11: 5 to

The next day I drew clocks on her magnetic board and asked

her to point to times as I said them, varying the form of the questions as much as possible.

'Which is the clock that says ten-fifteen? the clock that says a quarter to three? the clock that says three? two forty-five? six twenty-five? a quarter past ten? twenty-five past six?'

I asked her twenty-five questions and she got them all right. I drew some more figures on the board and asked her to point to the number of seconds in a minute, the number of minutes in an hour, the number of hours in a day, and so on. She got them all right.

That evening I decided to introduce Annie to an authority on mathematics, and I showed her a textbook on arithmetic by Hamlyn Greene, a beautifully written classic Victorian work.

I read the section on long multiplication to her quickly to explain a few unfamiliar words and stuck a photocopy of it on her cot for the night. The pages I had copied included multiplication tables. I did not read these out, and it was only when I was taking Annie back to the ward that I thought to ask her whether she knew multiplication tables. She responded 'Yes', and I gave her a quick test. I wrote 24, 72, 66, 84 on the board and asked her to point to 2 x 12, 12 x 7, 9 x 8, 6 x 4, 11 x 6, all of which she did quickly and accurately.

On Wednesday I worked out a long multiplication in front of her and then I set her 234 x 27. She worked on it by pointing to the number I was to write down, starting with the first number to the right of the top row. The board ended up as shown in Diagram 17.

Homework for Wednesday night was Hamlyn Greene on complex addition and subtraction. Annie's performance so far suggested that she knew about them already, but Hamlyn Greene expressed mathematics so elegantly that I thought she would enjoy reading him anyway.

Diagram 17

```
      234
   ×   27
    1638
    4680
    6318
```

1 2 3 4 5
 6 7 8 9 0

For the weekend I gave Annie this number line:

Diagram 18

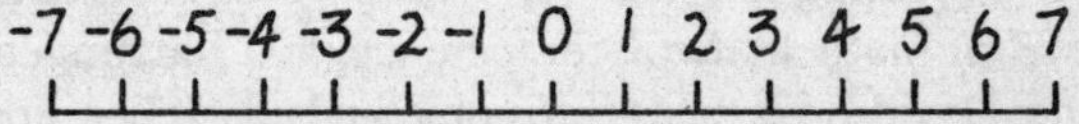

-7 -6 -5 -4 -3 -2 -1 0 1 2 3 4 5 6 7

I explained that each positive number had a corresponding negative number. I wanted to see if she could deduce unaided the rules for dealing with negative numbers. When I questioned her about them on Monday her answers showed that she had not got the principle involved, so I explained it to her using the number line. After that she answered correctly a string of questions: 2 - -2, -16 - -4, -2 x 2.

On Wednesday 29 June I explained that an unknown variable could be representated by x and gave her two simple questions for homework: if $27 - x = 23$, what is the value of x? and if $3x = 12$, what is the value of x?

They were easy questions, and she answered them

105

correctly on Monday. I set Annie a new sum: if $4x = 2y$ and $3x + 3y = 27$ what are the values of x and y? I wanted to introduce her to the concept of multiple variables. Several people criticized the sum as being too hard for her, but it did not seem too difficult to me, requiring only a logical mind and minimal mathematical knowledge. Annie answered it correctly when I asked her on Wednesday: $x = 3, y = 6$.

On 19 July I gave Annie a lesson on money. It sounds odd to teach her about dollars and cents after teaching her negative numbers, but she had lived all her life in an institution. She had never seen a full set of Australian currency, and had never touched on decimals. I mustered a full set of currency (excluding a $50 note), explained the relationship between dollars and cents, and in the process explained decimals. Then I set her two problems: what is the smallest number of coins making up 88 cents and what is the number of two-cent coins in $4.60? She got them both right.

I was beginning to sense that Annie would soon outstrip my level of mathematical competence, and I arranged for a friend, David Brownridge, to come and coach her. For six months Annie had extra mathematics lessons with David, which dealt with some of the fundamental concepts of mathematics and truth theory, and she went on having more basic lessons with me on practical subjects such as measurement, weight, and area.

ANNIE: I took longer to read a page then than now, but I could read anything I can read now. Some uncommon words I was still working out, but I could get every word I had ever heard spoken.

Being physically handicapped alters your expectations of time. You experience total inactivity for such long periods that you become skilful at filling them. During gaps in my life I vied with myself to try my brain against itself, calculating things which I knew existed but whose values I did not know. Being able to see the occasional television programme gave me some ideas. The Bronowski *Ascent of Man* programmes were critical in bringing me in contact with scientific method. In St Nicholas there was not much call for it, but it stopped me becoming intellectually barren. From them I was prepared to use mathematics.

When Joey taught us about fractions, suddenly everything started to come together. I started doing arithmetic for fun. I also tried to work out some constants. I had a go at the speed of light, using the distance of the moon from earth (which had been given coverage during the Apollo missions) and the stated delay time for radio signals. My calculation was unavoidably rough, because the time was to the nearest second. I made a stab at calculating the miles per second. I could not convert, because I had no idea how many feet there were in a mile.

Giving *pi* a value was impossible because I knew nothing about measurement. I could see that there was a relationship between the radius and the outside of circles. I did not know what it was called until later. Getting peak triangles (that is what I used to call two joined right-angle triangles) was easy in a hospital where everyone is in nappies. Bronowski covered Pythagoras, and I had ample opportunity to think about the implications. The hospital nappies were not square, and every time the nurses folded a nappy they had to square it first. I became aware of symmetry and its importance in geometry. To calculate I used a crude abacus based on the clock. I used to work in base twelve. I stored the units, treating them as minutes; the twelves I stored on the hour numbers and the grosses I stored on my cot bars.

A knowledge of mathematics rates high in my experience, as it enabled me to occupy myself happily for the later part of my time at St Nicholas. The best bit of work I did was in extrapolating multiplication and division from the addition and subtraction on *Sesame Street*. Multiplication seemed obvious: you added two sets of cot bars together and that meant two thirteens were twenty-six and likewise thirteen twos. Division was harder. I ruined a large part of a stupendous work on A-bombs because I could not divide properly.

Chapter Ten

By the middle of June Annie had managed to convince quite a number of people of her ability. But I was not entirely persuaded. At the back of my mind there was the fear that I might be subconsciously manipulating Annie's arm. I knew I was not doing it on purpose, but I had heard stories about teachers who wanted children to succeed so much that they 'produced' the success they were looking for. I didn't think I fell into that category. If I were manipulating her arm would I have chosen such an unflattering first sentence? Why was it that she could not spell as well as I could? And why were there times when we had misunderstandings and difficulties and could not communicate at all? But I still wondered, out loud, in front of Annie. I needed to find some way for Annie to communicate without my help.

Jean Vant, my old boss at St Nicholas, was by that time a lecturer at Burwood State Teachers' College, and on Tuesday 14 June she brought in Simon Haskell, a British authority on teaching physically handicapped people, to talk about some new equipment that Annie might be able to use to communicate independently. He told me about the Possum equipment that had been developed in Britain. The Possum equipment was based around a typewriter which the handicapped person could operate by pressing a switch when the wanted letter lit up on a grid containing letters and characters. The equipment meant that anyone able to control one movement consistently could have access to a typewriter keyboard and could work a calculator, heater, air-conditioner or television channel switch. It sounded marvellous.

By now Annie could read a book if I sat by her to turn the pages or if I bought two copies, pasted them up and stuck them on her cot bars.

After Annie had done her mathematics the next day she read *The Terrible Battle* from the Nippers series: twenty-three pages, approximately 1400 words. I was talking to someone else while she was reading it, and we had a lot of interruptions, but she signalled by making a noise when she wanted me to turn the page. I asked her comprehension questions on it, and she answered them correctly.

'Were there any words in the book you didn't know?', I asked.

'Yes.'

'Which ones?'

She spelt 'atte', and I went through the book looking for those letters. I had stopped her before she finished spelling and the word she was trying to spell was 'mattered'.

She did some more reading on Thursday morning. I chose *Mary Poppins* for her and propped it up on the table. I had some other children to work with, but every time I walked past Annie I turned over a page. Later I asked her some questions on the book. I was limited in the kinds of questions I could ask because of the speed at which she worked. I could hardly ask her for an outline of the plot; it would have taken hours. I had to ask her such things as 'What was the name of the old nurse?' and 'Mary Poppins said she would leave when something happened. What was it?'

I was checking comprehension, not spelling, and I stopped as soon as it was obvious that Annie knew the answers. She read fourteen pages, which was about 1600 words.

In the evening I brought Annie, with Mark and Angela,

to the playroom to read them *Where Babies Come From*, and I talked about their handicaps. I knew that they would all have heard quite a few theories discussed over their cots, and I wanted to talk about the causes of their handicaps with them frankly.

On Friday Annie came up to the playroom to do some more reading, but I did not have a chance to test her. In the evening I mounted *The Shrinking of Treehorn* on sheets of paper and stuck it on her cot for weekend reading. I always made an effort to put up plenty of reading or homework on Friday to give her something to do in the weekend if she was not coming home with us.

We were getting close to the date when the Superintendent wanted to see the videotape, and on Thursday evening we filmed some more of Annie's work with the help of Margot, one of the social workers. I set up Annie with her arm in the sling. Margot asked her a question whose answer she did not know.

'What kind of pet has Rosie?'

I worked the camera.

Margot was unable to interpret Annie's gestures. When Annie pointed to 'd', which was out of her reach, and made gestures indicating that she wanted the board moved, Margot did not understand. Annie switched her attack to 'pup'. Margot got one 'p', but then stopped coping. I shut off the camera in a rage, not at Margot or Annie, but at the doctors who had made this painful charade necessary.

Annie defused the situation by asking me to read her *Mary Poppins*.

On Friday we had a visit from David Brownridge. I was upset because the hospital Manager had just told me that I had to fire half my sessional staff. We had finally exhausted the accumulated child endowment funds, and there was not enough money to pay their wages.

David suggested that we go to the newspapers and

complain, but after a long discussion we decided against it.

The purpose of David's visit was to see if Annie could use Morse Code. To use it she would need to master an on-off-pause response. David wrote up the letters and their codes on the blackboard, and the table in front of Annie's pusher was divided into three segments: dot, dash, and pause. Annie had to move her hand from segment to segment, but it was no good. Her physical responses were simply not controlled enough, and her arm kept cramping.

We did not take Annie home for the weekend, but we came in to visit her on Sunday. On this occasion Chris tried out his pet communications scheme, which involved setting up the alphabet in frequency order and dividing the table in front of Annie into two sections, the left-hand side labelled 'yes' and the right-hand 'no'. The person working with Annie was to call the letters of the alphabet and Annie was to move her hand from 'no' to 'yes' if the letter indicated was the one she wanted. We got as far as 'talc' this way with some difficulty and then began to strike major problems. We went right through the alphabet without getting any response from Annie. I finally gave her the alphabet board and she finished off the sentence: 'Talc powder is nice.'

Chris asked Annie plaintively why his system did not work, and she spelt 'I am too slow.' When you called the letter she wanted she was unable to move before you had gone on to the next letter.

The biggest problem for Annie is in timing her responses. She can make a deliberate movement, but timing the movement is very difficult for her. If she makes an enormous amount of effort she can usually control her response quite well for a short time, but the effort required seems to exhaust her and she is then unable to respond at all. We might have got further if we had concentrated exclusively on one system. But I was still working with a large number of children, including ten who were communicating with me by spelling on the alphabet board or using the circles, and Annie had only a limited amount of time to communicate with me by any means. If I refused to allow her to communicate except by Morse Code or Chris's yes/no method she would have been lucky to spell out a sentence a week. At the time, it seemed perverse to cut back her communication although if I had known that we would still be fighting a battle two years later about her ability to communicate independently I may have opted for some other system.

We made the vital videotape on Tuesday 28 June. Annie had asked for Chris to come in, and he and Philip Graves were there. Chris and Philip asked the questions which were to be answered by Annie pointing, arm unsupported, to one of four answers written on her board. We all got very cross. Annie was co-operative, except when she was asked 'What are nine nines?' She preferred to answer the question, 'What is −5 − −5', and she pointed correctly to zero.

When Chris and Philip left, Annie and I looked at the tape together. It was rather disappointing, although her pointing was clear enough. The whole exercise had been dehumanizing for all of us.

On Wednesday afternoon I showed the videotape to an audience of doctors and senior staff at St Nicholas. The Superintendent said it was unconvincing. The nursing sister from Annie's ward, who had seen Annie working on the board on a number of occasions and had been there on the first day when Annie had pointed to objects, spoke up for her. Most of the staff just did not speak. I was aware that the videotape had defects: because there was only one camera you could never see Annie's face and hands together, so that if the camera showed where her hand was pointing you could not see where her eyes were looking and vice versa; and it was obviously a staged event which placed Annie under great stress. These problems were compounded because most of those present at the screening were doctors who were not used to working with athetoids. People who see the athetoid movement pattern regularly find it easy to discern the differences between intentional and non-intentional movements. Outsiders often find it difficult to see any distinction at all.

I suggested that rather than dissect the tape they come and see Annie for themselves. The Superintendent agreed but left without making a date. He did not see Annie use the alphabet board for another fifteen months. By the time the videotape was made, Mark and Angela were both using communications boards to 'talk' to two experienced teacher aides from the Department of Education, and neither had ever needed arm supports.

On Thursday 30 June Annie made a new friend. She was in the playroom reading when Philip Graves came in with Jean Melzer, a Senator in the Australian Parliament.

I asked Annie if she had heard of Senator Melzer.

'Yes', she responded, with a big smile.

'When?', I asked Annie.

Annie spelt out, 'Radio.'

Senator Melzer had been interviewed on the radio last Sunday.

ANNIE: Jean Melzer was the first visitor to see me spell. When I was asked how I knew her it was great to tell her about the interview I had heard her give. She had no doubt I was communicating, partly because Rosie was so embarrassed.

Chapter Eleven

Annie badly needed an independent means of communication to benefit from her new skills and to provide proof for the sceptics at the hospital. The next step was to learn what we could about the technology available for physically handicapped people.

On Friday 1 July we visited the Lincoln Institute, the Melbourne training centre for physiotherapists, speech therapists, and occupational therapists, to try out some equipment. We saw some very exciting things: typewriters and calculators operated by different means to suit people with all kinds of handicaps; things you could blow or suck or twitch or shout at; devices that let handicapped people use the telephone, or turn on the air-conditioning, or adjust the television.

We were looking for a page-turner so that Annie could read a book by herself. Staff at the institute showed us a very cunning device. To operate it you pushed a large, sensitive button and a small vacuum-cleaner swung around in front of the page that had been read and sucked it away from the pages behind it, and a slide moved around behind the page and pushed it over. We found that the touch-sensitive button could be set to respond to very small pressure. Annie operated it that day with both hands, her head, her foot, and her shoulder, all seemingly with equal ease.

We made an appointment to try the communications

module the following week and returned to St Nicholas elated. I took Annie to the playroom when we got back and scrambled some eggs for her dinner. I thought some celebration was in order after her efforts that afternoon. What we had seen certainly gave us cause for elation. Machines like these open up new horizons for handicapped people. Not only can they provide independent communication for people like Annie who are handicapped by their lack of speech, they can also provide the means for handicapped people to study, type, and earn a living. A handicapped person can now control anything that can be controlled electrically, and that covers everything from calculators to door locks. The technology for what we wanted was certainly there.

On Monday morning Annie and I discussed the Carbalinguaduc machines we had seen at the Lincoln Institute.

'How do you think you could best use the switch?', I asked. I thought she should use her hands, and she agreed.

'Which hand?', I asked.

She pointed to 'r'.

'What part of the hand?', I asked.

She spelt out 'thumb' and then 'I can yell.' She might be able to use the microphone input.

'Which piece of equipment do you want first, the page-turner or the Possum?', I asked her.

She spelt, 'I want a page-turner. Please arrange pension.'

It was the most realistic choice, and I was only worried that we would need the support of the Superintendent before we would be able to get it.

Although Annie was getting an invalid pension, and it was paid into a trust account bearing her name, the money was not at her disposal. If she asked for it to be spent in a particular way, her request would not necessarily be granted. The hospital could spend it 'on her behalf', without her consent, and some ludicrous purchases were made with her money. At one stage it was used to buy an enormous vinyl reclining armchair that Annie could not sit in.

I thought that there might be some problems about buying the page-turner, which cost about $1000, but when I took Annie's request to the Deputy Superintendent he said that she shouldn't have to pay for such a thing, that it should be bought by the hospital. He told me that if I put in a submission to buy it out of hospital funds he would arrange it.

I did as he suggested. My submission said, in part: 'As three children in St Nicholas can now read, and others are on the way, we need a page-turner.' It went through all levels of the administration without question, and was eventually passed by the three-man Mental Health Authority.

It still amazes me that nobody along the line took any apparent interest in the statement that three children in an institution for the profoundly retarded were able to read.

The page-turner is a wonderful machine, but its price illustrates the enormous cost of the auxiliary equipment that physically handicapped people need. None of it is available on medical benefits in Australia, and there are no assistance schemes. The assumption seems to be that this kind of equipment will be bought by people who have become incapacitated as a result of motor car accidents and who will have a lot of money from damages awarded to them to cover costs.

Annie's voracious appetite for books could not be contained until the page-turner arrived. Annie had chosen a new book, *The Man with the Shattered World*, one she had overheard me discussing with her volunteer helper, Kate Moore. I had noticed Annie jumping up and down in her pusher while we talked about the book.

'Do you want to read it?', I asked.

'Yes', she responded.

The book is a fascinating but difficult work on brain damage by the Russian psychologist, Luria, a case history of a man who had suffered extreme injuries to his brain from a war-time bullet wound. I could see that the subject would interest Annie greatly, but as I stuck some of his rather technical diagrams and descriptions on Annie's cot I wondered. If they did not baffle Annie, they were certainly going to baffle the ward staff.

On Monday evening I checked her comprehension. I drew a rough map of the brain and asked her to point to spots as I named them. Where a word like 'parietal' came up and I thought that she might have difficulty with its pronunciation, I spelt it as well as saying it. I asked her to show me the pons, frontal lobe, cerebellum, parietal lobe, medulla, and occipital lobe, all of which she was able to do correctly.

On Tuesday 5 July I chatted with Annie about uranium and nuclear power because of the news reports of anti-uranium demonstrations.

'Are you in favour of Australia's exporting uranium?', I asked.

'No', she responded, laughing.

'Only two bombs have ever been dropped on people deliberately. Do you know about them?', I asked.

'Yes', Annie replied.

'Do you know where they fell?', I asked.

Annie spelt out 'Hiro' and 'Nag' on the board.

I went on talking about the second world war, asking her an occasional question.

'What was the name of the British Prime Minister?'

'Chur.'

'The name of the German leader?'

'Hit.'

'The Italian leader?'

'Muss.'

'What was the large country that remained neutral until attacked by Germany?'

'Russ.'

'The name of the Chinese leader at the beginning of war?'
'Chia'.
'The name of the Chinese leader after the revolution?'
'Mao.'

Annie obviously knew a lot more about modern history than I had thought.

'Who,' I asked, 'do you think was the greatest person to have lived in the twentieth century?' I told her it did not have to be a politician, it could be an artist or writer or whatever she wanted.

She spelt, 'Einstein.'

The next day my lecturer from the literacy course at Melbourne State Teachers' College, Joy Peletier, came to the hospital to check on the progress of my project, which was based on Annie.

I had mentioned Annie during our seminars, and the class was asking eagerly each week for the latest bulletin. This was the first time Joy had met Annie.

In Joy's presence I checked Annie's homework: some simple simultaneous equations, which she got right without any trouble. I explained to Joy about David Brownridge coming in to coach Annie. Annie spelt out, 'When will I do mathematics?', and I told her that it would probably be from 5 to 7 two nights a week. Annie was very excited and spelt out, 'I like to see *Sesame Street*!' It runs from 4.30 to 5.30 and I had forgotten about it completely. I told her we would ask David to come at 5.30 instead.

I was talking to Joy about *Sesame Street* when Annie indicated that she would like to join in. She spelt 'I like s' and I jumped in, 'Oh, you're going to spell "I like *Sesame Street*" aren't you? Point to the 's' for Street if that's right and I'll let you off the rest.' She pointed to the 's', looking highly aggrieved, and then swung her arm around with a big grin and erased it.

By this time we had established a method of erasure that

worked extremely well. When Annie pointed to a letter I said it aloud; if the letter was not the one she wanted she would move her hand off the board to the right, and I would 'erase' the last letter or word I had said. If I was not sure which letter she was pointing to I did not say anything, and she had to point again and again until she did it clearly.

Her next letter was clear enough. After erasing the 's' she pointed to the 'a' and went on until she had spelt out, 'I like saying things.' It was true. Annie liked saying things for herself. If anyone guessed too early, before the answer was inevitable, Annie would go to some pains to alter what she was going to say, sometimes getting herself into a mess in the process.

On Thursday 7 July I took part, with the permission of the authorities, in a paediatricians' study group at the Queen Victoria Medical Centre, with at least two professors among those present. The subject of the meeting was Anne McDonald. Dr Philip Graves introduced me and I presented Annie's case history, explained how I had taught her to communicate, being careful to describe the method I was using and the amount of support I had to give her, and I told them how far she had gone.

After the reactions I had got at St Nicholas I was prepared for disbelief, but nobody present questioned that I was truthful and that this kind of thing was possible.

As Annie had been 'confined to barracks' last weekend, we made sure we took her home this time. We did a lot of activities, but the most important thing that happened was a mistake. Chris asked Annie what kind of music she liked because he wanted to know what kinds of records to put on when she was home. Annie spelt 'mist.'

'Was it the name of a group?, the name of a song?', I asked.

'No.' An embarrassed Annie corrected it to 'most'.

We laughed at her for having made such an elementary

mistake or, rather, for having allowed my misinterpretation to go unchallenged.

It was a small incident, but it provided the evidence that was to convince me that Annie was able to communicate, and that I was not subconsciously manipulating or influencing her in any way.

On Tuesday 12 July, Dot Chandler, one of the social workers based at the hospital and someone who had worked for me some time before as a part-time playleader, came to see what Annie was doing. I spent some time telling Dot about people believing I was moving Annie's arm.

Dot was interested in supporting Annie's arm herself, and Annie said she was prepared to try it. Dot held her arm while Annie spelled out, 'You laughed at mist.' I had not mentioned Saturday's incident to Dot, and she had no way of knowing about it.

When I realized how important the sentence was I asked Annie if she had just made any sentence or whether she had chosen one that Dot would not understand. She spelt, 'I chose it.' She knew that I would have written Saturday's sentence in the diary I was keeping.

Dot was very pleased to have been the agent for Annie to provide proof that she was communicating independently of the people supporting her, but it did not alter Dot's view of Annie's communication. Having listened to me and watched Annie spelling, Dot had believed in Annie's ability to communicate before the 'mist' incident proved it. This was important. As Annie said much later, because Dot believed in her to start with, it meant that she did not have to worry about Dot's reaction if the attempts at communication failed. Annie was less tense with Dot than when she was being 'tested'.

Dot and I talked about some of the other hospital children. I asked Annie if she knew who the other bright children were in Ward 4. She said 'Yes', and spelt out four sets of initials. Dot mentioned Shirley, a girl we had both worked with, not one of the Beanbaggers. Dot thought Shirley might be bright, but I said that Shirley was more physically able than the other children, and it misled you into thinking she was brighter. I did not think she was intelligent at all. Annie jumped up and down at this, an indication that she wanted to say something, and when I gave her the board she spelt, 'Shirley is always underrated.' Shirley is now a fully literate Beanbagger.

We wound up the session at 9.30, and I put Annie to bed. Dot drove me home, and Chris showed her my diary entry for last Saturday.

I thought that from here on it would be plain sailing: Dot would be able to go to the Superintendent of St Nicholas and tell him about the incident that made it quite clear that Annie was communicating independently of me. Then everything would start to fall into place.

I was relieved. Anybody who helps a handicapped person communicate must wonder how much they are putting into that communication. I knew I was not moving Annie's arm deliberately, whatever people thought. What I did not know was whether I was subconsciously manipulating her, or imagining her hand movements over the letters and making up sentences to fit what were really random twitchings.

Dot did not know about the 'mist' incident, and therefore she could not have manipulated Annie's arm to spell out the sentence about it. The only logical conclusions were that Annie had learnt to spell and could communicate independently of the person supporting her arm.

The proof was very important in the development of my relationship with Annie. She had been aware that I was not entirely confident about her abilities. In distrusting myself I was also distrusting her. But I could not treat her as an intelligent communicating sixteen-year-old until I was sure that she was communicating. It must have been hard for Annie to relax and be confident with someone who doubted her, however marginally.

The proof also stiffened my backbone in the battles that followed.

Nothing will rival the excitement of my first few sessions with Annie, but that night I was almost as happy.

ANNIE: Too many teachers are afraid of their students making them appear foolish. Perhaps this was Rosie's greatest strength – she never cared what anyone said as long as she thought she was right. Until we laughed at 'mist' Rosie could not be sure I was communicating independently. However, she gave me a chance regardless. If she had not I would still be in St Nicholas, if I was still alive.

Chapter Twelve

Dot Chandler went to the Superintendent to tell him about her session with Annie. She was given what had become the usual response. He greeted her story with polite disbelief. People who said that they thought my claims about the children were right were told that they must be mistaken. The position was extraordinary. Because I could not prove that the children could communicate, nobody in authority was prepared to come and see them communicate. Until I could prove that they were intelligent nobody would come and assess them. Guilty until proved innocent. The children were profoundly and hopelessly retarded until they could prove they were intelligent.

The Superintendent was not alone. People working in the Mental Health Authority whom I had heard espouse radical ideas on the care of the handicapped could not face the idea that I could be right. It was simply too threatening; my discovery questioned the basic assumptions on which care was offered in institutions.

In St Nicholas, the Superintendent's attitude had two effects: junior staff members were reluctant to be seen to side with someone who had displeased those in power, and senior staff members were reluctant to do anything about the children in the face of the Superintendent's opposition. But my relations with the ward assistants were still friendly.

I approached Dr David Barlow, the Director of Mental Retardation Services, who agreed to organize a group of professionals from outside St Nicholas to assess the children. The Superintendent nominated Jean Vant, a lecturer from Burwood State Teachers' College, to the assessment panel. Jean had been chief psychologist for the Mental Health Authority and, of course, she was my old boss.

Jean Vant made her first visit on Thursday 1 August 1977, and she arrived just after Annie had started her mathematics lesson with David Brownridge. I suggested that Annie spell something with me supporting her arm to show Jean how she was able to communicate. Annie spelt out, 'As test ask something about David.'

We decided that Jean should support Annie's arm while I asked her questions.

'Does David have a car?', I asked.

'No.'

Jean was having difficulty in supporting Annie's arm.

'What is the name of David's girl friend?' Her name was Carmel.

Annie tried to reach 'c' and in her effort hit all the letters around it. Annie was very tense, and Jean, like other people, was having an exhausting time fighting against Annie's spasm. Nobody said 'c' was correct, so Annie dived for 'k'. Jean called it. Annie pointed to 'a' clearly enough and then we gave up.

I went to make coffee, and Jean went on to the next stage of the test. She showed Annie a photograph of a child, told her his name, and asked her to tell me. When I returned Annie fooled about. She spelt 'Tobias', which was wrong, and according to Jean flirted with the correct letters by pointing to letters that were one off the correct ones. I could tell from feeling Annie's arm that she was fooling around and that she had chosen the letters deliberately. I was very angry. I blasted Annie for her lack of co-operation and I took her straight back to the ward. I told her that if anything happened to me before she had proved that she could communicate she would be abandoned in St Nicholas for ever. I felt bad about putting pressure on her in that way, but I knew my statements were true.

When I brought Annie to the playroom to read next morning she spelt, 'I am sorry about Alistair.' I checked with Jean. Alistair was the name of the boy in the photograph.

Next time Jean came she brought a comprehension piece for Annie to read and answer questions on. We decided that Annie would read it when I was out of the room and I would return and support her arm while she answered questions on it.

Annie did not perform very well. She seemed tired, and she appeared to want to say other things. The answer to one of the questions was 'gin'. When Annie had got as far as 'gi' Jean made the mistake of saying, 'Oh, I know what's coming next.' Annie spelt out 'gift', which although not incorrect was not as precise. We ran out of time. Later I went through the list of questions with Annie, and she fooled around again. I was angry.

The next day I tried again. I was feeling guilty about the day before. I rationalized that personal relationships were more important to Annie than test results, and that she was trying out the situation. I thought that she wondered how far I would go. Would I still like her if she did not perform? Was I only interested in her as a display object?

I told Annie that she did not have to answer the questions if she did not want to, but I was hoping that she would.

She began by spelling 'Leo is beaut' which referred to Dr Leo Murphy who had come to the hospital with Jean Vant. When I accepted that without complaint she went on to answer the questions. She spelt, 'Jean's friend is called Ginnie.' The correct answer was Annie; the passage had been a humorous one about a person with a drinking problem.

Annie was still testing me. She spelt 'She got the gin from unnuity', obviously a stab at 'annuity'. Where she had come across the word I do not know. Jean had not used the word, but it was a good answer.

On Friday 12 August Annie was the subject of a case conference at St Nicholas. She was not present. Jean Vant gave the Superintendent a preliminary report on her assessments. It read:

I am satisfied that Annie is very much aware of her surroundings and can respond to them. She was given a passage to read whose contents were known only to Dr Murphy and myself, then three typed questions relating to it. One answer was given in my presence, and although not the one expected was quite appropriate. However, I am not basing my judgement solely on this but also on her observed behaviour, her expressive response to people being very readable and indicating a degree of sophistication incompatible with severe retardation. Until a more satisfactory method is found to enable her to communicate I do not think one can be specific about the extent of her ability. I would think that Annie and one or two of the other children (or rather young adults) could learn to use the Possum typewriter, which would greatly extend their possibility of communicating and therefore enable us to be surer in our judgement.

I was then quizzed about the exact level of the passage that Annie had read. What was in question was whether Annie was profoundly retarded. If she was able to read no more than 'The cat sat on the mat' that would negate the previous diagnosis.

I gave the shortest report I could. I said I had started trying to develop a system of communication with Annie four months ago and that she was now fully literate. I left the rest of the story to unfold through questions.

The Deputy Superintendent listed all the points against Annie on a blackboard. They were her lack of head control, her incontinence (this when she was living in a ward with no toilets), and the ward staff's inability to read her homework.

I asked the Superintendent if the hospital would buy a Possum machine to help the children communicate. He said there were no problems and of course we could have one.

He gave a strong warning about the possibility of damaging headlines in *Truth*, a weekly Melbourne muck-raking newspaper. No one, he said, should say that Annie was of normal intelligence.

'In that case,' I replied, 'I will confine myself to saying that Annie is brighter than I am, and people can take that as they like.'

I meant what I said. Four months of working with Annie, watching how fast she learnt, and how far she had educated herself under almost impossible circumstances had convinced me that she was intelligent.

It was a satisfactory case conference. It would have been gratifying if people had agreed that Annie was intelligent and could communicate, but we did not expect that, and we were not terribly disappointed when they did not say it. But we badly needed an independent means of communication for Annie, and we had been offered a Possum typewriter.

Immediately after the meeting I wrote a submission to the Health Commission on the need for a Possum typewriter at St Nicholas. I said: 'There are now three children at St Nicholas who are communicating very laboriously by spelling, and another seven are well on the way towards this.' The submission was signed by the Education Department's head teacher and me, and was accepted by the Health Commission without question. None of the people who read it bothered to investigate it; nobody realized that if what it said was correct then more would be required for the children than the purchase of a Possum.

By August 1977 ten children were using communications boards, and I was spending an enormous amount of time on the telephone trying to get money for equipment or help for them. I tried many avenues. I rang the Department of Social Security, the Royal Children's Hospital, the state Health Department, the Handicapped Person's Information Centre, the federal Department of Health, private charities and many more.

This was just the beginning of a list that grew steadily longer and a response that became increasingly more depressing. Everybody was interested in my work but nobody had any help to offer. The St Nicholas children fell outside any of the standard categories. They were not living at home with their parents, so none of the systems for helping parents applied. Because voluntary agencies are geared for parents who keep their children at home, they provide very limited accommodation. Because the children in my group had been injured through no fault of their own, there was no insurance money for them. Again and again I came up against the same brick wall: government care for children who cannot live with their parents falls into two areas in Victoria: children who are not handicapped are the responsibility of the Department of Social Welfare, and children who are severely handicapped in any way come under the care of the Mental Health Authority. In practice this means they are all put in institutions for the mentally retarded.

The state does not make a particularly good parent. A child who lives at home is able to go to an outpatients' department of a public hospital and have a wheelchair prescribed without cost. A child in St Nicholas does not go to an outpatients' department and does not get a wheelchair, or special boots, or any other special equipment. The St Nicholas children are kept alive but that is the end of it.

As well as searching for help from outside organizations I lobbied inside the Mental Health Authority. Dr David Barlow, the Director of Mental Deficiency Services was very sympathetic. He mentioned the need for independent proof of the children's abilities, but he was aware of the 'Catch 22': the children would find it difficult to provide convincing proof without the therapy and the equipment they would not get until they had provided convincing proof. He said he did not think there would be money to move the children until 1978 or 1979. I thought he was being intolerably pessimistic.

By the end of 1979 there were still eleven intellectually normal children in a hospital for the profoundly retarded, and there was still no equipment.

St Nicholas's other dilemmas intervened and took my mind off the problems of Annie and her friends. I was faced by the need to sack some staff because the hospital's child endowment funds were exhausted. I was still doing work for my Diploma of Education, and Chris did not see much of me except at weekends. He was getting morose.

In September Jean Vant came to see Annie and some of the other children to make a fuller report. Her report on Anne said:

I have observed her working with the magnetic letter board both as the person supporting her and the person who was asking the questions. I am satisfied in both instances that she did indeed answer the questions and in each case had read the material and the questions.

This report, from a person who had been the Mental Health Authority's Senior Psychologist, should have put the matter beyond doubt.

The Superintendent's reaction was characteristic. When he spoke to me in October about the report he said it showed that Anne McDonald was 'a tiny bit more intelligent' than he had thought. Otherwise he ignored it. Later he said that he did not believe Jean Vant. It was the recurrent problem: as soon as anyone said that they supported me they lost their credibility.

It was the same with the other professionals who supported my views on the children. They had nothing to gain by supporting me: they would get no credit from any of the children's achievements and no blame if the children remained intellectual blanks. They were only saying what they believed to be the truth. As soon as they did so, they were forced into an adversary role. They could then do one of three things. They could retract, and say that they had been mistaken. They could stick to what they had said but ignore the implication, or they could fight to have their belief accepted as the truth. Nobody took the first course. One or two took the second. Most of the people who had grounds for believing me stayed in to fight, despite the problems this created for them later.

Dr Murphy passed on Jean's second report to some senior members of the Mental Health Authority outside St Nicholas. For a brief moment it seemed as if somebody would act on it. Dr Barlow called me over to his office and told me that he had spoken to top staff in Mental Health about it, and they were stunned but excited. They had asked him to tell me that they would give me any help in their power and that I was to give him a list of the things I needed. I gave him one on the spot: a Possum, an occupational therapist, a physiotherapist, wheelchairs, and another teacher. And that was the last I heard of that.

Shortly afterwards I was demoted and it was strongly suggested that I resign from St Nicholas. Demotion is not quite the right word. I was already a ward assistant, the lowest position and the lowest-paid one in the hospital, but I did have my title of play-leader removed, and I was no longer to be in charge of the department I had founded. A kind of petty harassment set in. I was not to be paid for any overtime. This was no problem because I had not been paid for overtime for some time. Instead I had taken time off in lieu to attend lectures for my course. Then I was told that I could not take time off in lieu. I would have to take time for my lectures as leave without pay. I agreed to do so, and continued to work after hours on a voluntary basis. Suddenly a number of previously unknown restrictions on voluntary work were brought into effect. I was told that I would have to apply one month in advance if I wanted to work late, specifying in my application the children concerned and the exact times I would be working with them. It did seem an unusually pedantic approach to an attempt to give a short-staffed hospital the benefit of a little unpaid labour. I was eventually allowed to resume voluntary work, but not until a number of battles had been fought.

After six months of procrastination I lost patience with the Mental Health Authority and I put in a submission to the Schools Commission, a federal body which handed out funds for a wide range of educational projects. I hoped that it would be interested in funding a really innovative project: the provision of 24-hour educational programmes for a group of children who had missed out, by my calculations, on about a hundred years of schooling between them. I proposed to give the children a year in which to achieve independent communication and to develop enough in other areas to be given reliable assessments of their intellectual functioning and their potential at the end of the year. Now I think I underestimated the time it would take. My purpose was best expressed in the dictum I wrote on the title page of my submission: 'If we keep handicapped people alive, we must give them a life worth living.' The submission was a large and elaborate document and said in part:

Literacy for these children is not just an academic achievement, giving them access to books, education and jobs. For the first time in their lives they have a chance to join the human race. Until they started in this programme not one of these children had communicated with anyone, ever. They had lain on their backs on mats on the floor for up to twelve years with no way of ever making their wishes known, of ever indicating that they had wishes, treated as babies because 'they can't walk, they can't talk – how can they be intelligent?'. They have suffered frustrations, deprivations and miseries impossible for us to imagine. Some day they will tell us what it was like.

Surprisingly, the children don't seem to be bitter. They are not the psychotic wrecks you might expect. Instead they are a cheerful group who get on well with each other and with me. They are incredibly gutsy, when you consider the extent of their physical handicaps – they try and keep on trying to do whatever physical task I set them. Fortunately they are able to see the funny side of the situations their handicaps land them in. Their eagerness to learn and their wide interests make them a delight to work with. The older children feel responsibility towards each other, and towards the world outside – one of the first sentences Annie spelt out was 'Note errors in my writing, Rosie, so we teach others.' Of course, the kids are not a bunch of Pollyannas – they can be miserable, and they can be completely bloody-minded – but they are certainly no worse than normal children, and I suspect they're better.

Right now the children are not interested in the past but in the future. They know I am making this submission, and they know why, and you should have seen the smiles on their faces when I told them. They need something to hope for – some of them were very discouraged when changes weren't made immediately their abilities became obvious. It is hard to explain that people don't want to believe it, that they don't want to see it, and that they hope it's all a mistake I've made. For the people who have been involved with these children over the years the truth is too uncomfortable to be easily accepted. I can understand this, but it's harder for the kids to. These children have been imprisoned since birth, firstly within their own bodies and secondly within the institution in which they live. It is not simply their education that depends on this submission, it is their whole lives. No child should ever have to justify its existence, but that is just what has been forced on these children. We distinguish ourselves from animals by our ability to communicate. These children are having to beg to be allowed to communicate. There is surely no human right more basic than this.

The submission included as an appendix a list of the children on whose behalf the submission was being made, their dates of birth, and their dates of admission to St Nicholas. I made the mistake of giving a copy of it to the Superintendent. The upshot was a letter that said:

The disclosure by you to an unauthorized body of names of the patients at St Nicholas is a serious breach of confidentiality. You are hereby warned that should there be a repetition of this offence appropriate action will be taken under public service regulations. Retain one copy of this memo for your information and sign and return the other copy in acknowledgment of its receipt.

He need not have worried: all we ever got back from the Education Department was a roneoed letter of rejection.

Putting in that submission to the Schools Commission made things much worse for me at St Nicholas, and for a few weeks I was the local pincushion. After a particularly torrid couple of days Annie spelt out, 'Leave St Nicholas. Children are not your responsibility', and it broke me up completely. It was a mad, noble gesture, probably no sooner made than regretted. I was Annie's lifeline; telling me to go was the equivalent of deciding to kill herself in a peculiarly painful and extended manner.

ANNIE: I meant it when I told Rosie to leave, but I would have been heartbroken if she had gone. Timidity is not her problem, fortunately, because she was attacked on all sides. Once the nurses saw that she was out of favour, she was made the punching-bag for everybody.

Chapter Thirteen

I began to worry about what would happen to the children if something happened to me. Most of them had nobody else whom they could communicate to or through, and there was very little documentation on any of the children except Anne, and that would be brushed aside if I were not there to lend it weight.

What worried me was the possibility of being sacked, having an accident, or becoming ill. Whatever the cause of my leaving, the effect would be the same.

In November 1977 I decided to try and set up a committee of those professionals working in the area who had had some direct contact with the children and believed that what I said about them was correct. They could provide back-up for me while I was at St Nicholas and back-up for the children if anything happened to me.

As usual, Annie was ahead of me. She had been very tense for a few days, and when I asked her to tell me what was troubling her, she spelt, 'I worry about you leaving. What would happen to us? Kill me first.' I reassured Annie by saying that if anything happened to me, Chris and the committee would continue to work on behalf of the children.

Everybody I approached about forming a committee agreed without hesitation. Because my group was known around the hospital as the Beanbaggers, the committee called itself the 'Beanbaggers Support Group'. It was a cosy enough title, but for a body that was asking governments for large sums of money it lacked dignity, and in 1979 its name was change to DEAL (Dignity, Education, and Language – A New Deal for the Handicapped).

In 1980 DEAL is a much larger organization with an elected committee, which consists of a paediatrician, a speech therapist, a social worker, a psychologist, a sociologist, a research assistant, two people who have experience in work with the handicapped, and two people with cerebral palsy.

Originally the committee was made up largely of those professionals who had found their reports on the children rejected out of hand by the Mental Health Authority. A letter went to the Authority at the end of January 1978, signed by an educationalist, two psychologists, and a paediatrician. It said in part:

Enclosed is an abridged version of the submission made by Ms Crossley to the Schools Commission in 1977.

We have seen all the children concerned in the submission, and some of us have seen a smaller number in depth. It is our belief that the claims made are true.

If this is so these children are owed a great deal by the community. They are owed an opportunity to show their potential by being provided with an optimal emotional and educational environment. In addition an immediate and continuing assessment is needed. The Mental Health Authority is best placed to do all this.

Whilst there is no doubt that these children have suffered greatly it is not easy or helpful to identify any person at fault. But now that they have succeeded in communicating their potential we consider that it is wrong to deny them a full assessment and a better environment without delay.

We are also concerned about the children's parents, most of whom have no idea of the claims being made for their children. We feel it would be in the best interests of all concerned if they could be brought into the discussions at this early stage.

The support I got from the committee was important to me,

and it may have something to do with my not being peremptorily fired. When it came to getting the message over to the Health Commission, however, it fared no better than I had, despite the undisputed professional expertise of its members. The Mental Health Authority heard nothing it did not want to hear.

Earlier it had been reported that Sir John Kerr, the Governor-General who had dismissed the Prime Minister, Gough Whitlam, in 1975, was about to retire. Annie, whose sympathies were all with the Labor Party, asked me then, 'Has Kerr another job?' I asked her if she had anything in mind, and she spelt 'Mental Health chairman.' I could see what she meant.

Before 1979 only one attempt was made to assess my claims that thirteen children at St Nicholas could spell. For obvious reasons, it had to be done in a scientific and clinical atmosphere.

Dr Roger Wales, a Reader in Psychology at the University of Melbourne, had volunteered to try and find a method of assessing the children that would not involve my participation. His method was admirably objective, involving videotaping the children as they made choices from pairs of words presented by another psychologist. The assessment of the responses was made later by groups of outsiders who knew neither the children nor the correct answers. We only got as far as pilot testing, but the results were promising. They suggested that 'the children are capable of performing better than their motor skills might lead us to believe ... they have given some indication of an ability to read and obey fairly complex instructions.'

As the tests were done in early 1978, and as most of the group had first been introduced to the alphabet less than six months before, I was not disappointed, even though the children's distrust of outsiders meant that the results were not as clear-cut as they might have been.

Annie, for example, agreed to do the test, and answered the first couple of questions correctly, but she was not enthusiastic and she worked very slowly. I think she resented being given such basic questions, and when Dr Wales ticked her off she got every other question quickly and confidently wrong. As Dr Wales pointed out, such a consistent error rate was unlikely to come about by chance, and it implied strongly that she knew the correct answers. The Mental Health Authority paid no attention to Dr Wales's findings.

Proof of the children's ability to communicate appeared in ordinary, everyday situations. Ann, a voluntary worker, asked Noelene, another of the Beanbaggers, which book she would like read to her. With Ann supporting her arm Noelene spelled *Peter Pun* [sic]. Ann looked through the bookshelf in the activities room, could not find the book and thought she must have misunderstood Noelene. Ann did not know that I was reading it to the group as a bedtime story and kept the copy in the ward dormitory.

I remember the surprise on the face of Angela's sister when at Angela's prompting I asked her about the Rod Stewart record she had got for Christmas. Likewise, the nurse in charge of the ward was surprised when I told her that Phillip, another member of the Beanbaggers group, had said that Ellie, his volunteer helper, had left a radio in the office for him; we had to search high and low to find it, but he was right.

Mark and Angela went on a camp with the Education Department teachers, who did not believe that they could communicate, and when they returned I asked the teacher-in-charge to ask Angela a question about the camp. Angela was asked whom they had met on the way to camp. I had not gone to the camp and did not know the answer. She spelt out 'Mum', which turned out to be correct. I suggested to Mark that he tell me something that the teachers had been up to at the camp. He spelt 'Dope.'

This incident may go some way towards explaining the general disquiet that the children's communication aroused. There is no doubt that you act more carefully in front of people who can tell on you later than in front of people you think cannot.

On one level my work with Annie was convincing enough. Most of the people who saw her working found it easy enough to believe, from her concentration, her eye movements, and the way she struggled to hit the letters, that the messages that came out were her own. Unfortunately this kind of evidence was not accepted. It was not even regarded as relevant.

On another level, unbiased proof of Annie's ability to communicate was rejected.

Soon Annie stopped being willing to perform tests that were designed to test my integrity. It was not a rational response, but it seemed to me to be linked to something central to her personality. She would not perform such a test to please me. She would not do it although her refusal would publicly embarrass me. She would not do it to save herself or to help others. The trouble was that the tests were designed to remove the possibility of my dishonesty, and if I was dishonest it would imply the annihilation of her personality. If I had been manipulating her, she was profoundly retarded. Annie was no longer prepared to have that put even as a hypothetical proposition.

It became clear that Annie would only co-operate in tests if she had a chance of putting in something of her own, if she could tell you something you did not know, or show you that she knew something you did not suspect she knew. Annie would do tests that were tests of her ability or knowledge but not tests whose only purpose was to check on my honesty.

Another reason Annie had for disliking tests was that she felt proof could be obtained more simply and more definitively by giving her access to various electronic communication devices. Before going to the Lincoln Institute to try the Carbalinguaduc she spelt, 'A demonstration is possible Friday.' She did not get a chance or try the communications equipment on that visit, but a week later a demonstration model of the Possum was brought to St Nicholas.

By twisting her shoulder against a micro-switch Annie was able to type 'ged ap'. She confirmed later that what she had been trying to say was 'Get a Possum.'

The day the Possum was delivered to the hospital in February 1978 she spelt, 'This could be the last time': the last time she would use the alphabet board. Unfortunately the Possum was out of order when it arrived, did not have some of the refinements of the demonstration model, and has been waiting to be repaired since April 1978.

Even so, mechanical faults were not our main problem. Because it was so important to me to have a clear demonstration of Anne's abilities, and because Anne had so desperately wanted independent communication, we had both glossed over the difficulties involved.

For quite a long time I continued to over-rate the degree of control Annie had over her movements. Before we got on to the machines we had tried a few alternative systems, and we had found that Annie was not able to move fast enough to use them. She could operate her page-turner well enough by hitting a switch; it did not matter how long she took to hit it as long as she had the patience to keep trying. It was a different matter to be able to hit a button just when a moving light paused on a panel of letters, when timing and reaction time were vital.

I lacked knowledge in the area. Working in mental health had separated me from the people working on this sort of equipment with physically handicapped children, and I was not allowed to ask for help. If we had been given the therapists I had asked for things would probably have been different. As it was we got almost nowhere.

A number of the children, including Annie, typed out short messages successfully on the Possum, although there were a large number of errors and consequent erasures; however, as we had no proper seating to steady the children, no switch-holders to steady the switches, no therapists to guide us, and a partially defective machine, the messages were only recorded with an adult holding the switch for the child to use. As we were trying to produce a result that could not be written off as human error or fraud, it was no help.

When Annie realized this she was upset, and she became depressed and reluctant to use the Possum at all. I found that I was also very tense, wound up by all that depended on the Possum. My tension communicated itself to the children and increased their tension, and that made it still more difficult to work with the machine. It was a relief to us all when the Possum was finally taken out of commission.

Towards the end of 1977, Melbourne State College, the place where I was working for my Diploma of Education and the state's major teacher training centre, showed sufficient faith in Annie to ask for permission to make a videotape of Annie and me working together. The idea was to show future students how even a very handicapped person could be taught to read and write when the motivation and the intelligence were there. The Superintendent of St Nicholas gave his permission, and we made the videotape on 13 December 1977, in the State College studio.

Annie was very enthusiastic. I told her that the tape was going to be shown to student teachers, and I asked her to think of something appropriate and short to say to them. I was particularly rigorous about her pointing during this session, refusing to accept any letters unless they were completely clear. This meant that Annie had to point to some characters four or five times before I said them aloud. She was very nervous but very determined, and the final result was very convincing. What she spelt was 'Too many tests.

Not enough teachers.' Because the tape was being made by professionals with multiple cameras it did not suffer in the same way that our home-made efforts had. The final tape was an hour long: half an hour of Annie spelling out the sentence and half an hour of my explaining the processes by which she had learnt to do it. It was quite impressive.

The Superintendent did not choose to view this videotape until 1979.

ANNIE: Communication is the most essential use to which spelling should be devoted. It should not be used as a test or an exhibition piece. Try being confined to a sentence a week and see how you feel about using that sentence to answer some stupid question about whether you live in St Nicholas. If Rosie had spent all her time giving tests we would not have had time to use spelling for our own communication. Crushing the personalities of speechless individuals is very easy: just make it impossible for them to communicate freely.

Chapter Fourteen

Anne's venturing into the outside world brought its own problems. St Nicholas was not ideal but at least there the reactions of the staff were predictable and you knew where you were with them. As she developed Annie was like a snail crawling away from its shell. Thirteen years in a maximum security institution had left her without any armour when she was away from the institution. The defence mechanisms she had developed so skilfully were designed to enable her to survive in an institution; they were not very helpful for her when she was outside it.

In 1975, when staff at St Nicholas went on strike and parents were asked to take their children home, the *Age* thought Annie's departure from the hospital significant enough for a front page story. It said:

Anne McDonald, a fourteen-year-old girl totally incapacitated by mental retardation and weighing only three stone [19 kilograms], will leave hospital for the first time in eleven years tomorrow because of the strike by psychiatric nurses.

The television cameras were waiting outside St Nicholas gates to film her departure.

What Anne had to contend with in the outside world were the prejudice and ignorance resulting in part from descriptions published in newspapers and on television of handicapped people. Several of her early experiences in 1977 will illustrate the problem.

One Saturday morning we went off to the Queen Victoria Market, Melbourne's big produce market. It is always packed on Saturdays with people buying their week's groceries, and Anne did not seem comfortable or happy.

After lunch we asked her why. She spelt 'The stars', hovering over the 'i' for a long time after the 'a'. She meant 'the stares'. People, and particularly children, did stare at Annie, there was no doubt about it, but the stares were not necessarily unfriendly. I suggested that attack was probably the best form of defence. If she stared back, she would probably find that most people stopped looking. I said she should not be too self-conscious. At places like the Victoria Market there are quite a number of more or less funny-looking people and everybody stares at everybody else. She was going to have to realize that not all the stares were directed at her and she would have to get used to crowded places.

When we took Annie back to the hospital after a weekend with us at the beginning of September she cried unconsolably for a long time. She was very depressed on Monday and Tuesday, did not want to leave the ward to take part in activities, and would not tell me what was upsetting her. I finally took her upstairs on Wednesday morning and told her that she must tell me what was wrong if she could. She spelt out, 'I affect kids badly.' Questioning elicited that this referred to an incident on our Sunday walk. I had not even noticed it. Without wanting to minimize the problems, I told Annie that people tend to take you at your own valuation. If you smile, look confident, stare back, you do better. I mentioned my webbed fingers, which could have been a source of difficulty with other children when I was at school if I had tried to hide them. Instead I treated them as something to show off, and it ended up with every other child in the class wishing that they had webbed fingers too. I also made the obvious points about bad manners. I emphasized the difference betweeen the reactions of people who had met her and those of strangers, and pointed out that it is acceptance by friends and family that really matters.

Annie was coming home with us almost every weekend now, and as usual next Saturday we collected her from the hospital. We picked her up at about three, came home, gave her an egg flip, and went for a walk on North Melbourne hill. When we got back Chris showed Annie a review in the *Melbourne Times*, a free local weekly paper, of *Baal*, one of Brecht's early plays, which was being performed by the Australian Performing Group in the headquarters of an alternative theatre in nearby Carlton. Chris asked Annie if she wanted to go. He was going in any case, and I said that I would go if Annie said yes. The review did not make it sound very entertaining, but it was being directed by James McCaughey, and he had been responsible for some of Melbourne's most interesting small theatre productions in the last few years. Annie said she did want to go, so Chris rang the theatre and booked some seats. We collected and paid for our tickets. At the door to the theatre, we were met by James McCaughey who told us that no babies were allowed. I told him Annie was not a baby. He repeated that babies were not allowed and we had an argument. James agreed to let us in if we guaranteed Annie's good behaviour and silence, which we did. Annie's public behaviour had always been exemplary, and she was as aware of the standard social requirements as any ordinary sixteen-year-old.

The theatre was set up with tiers of seats around a central playing area, and as James was being unco-operative we had to lift Annie's pusher up to the top tier. The play started almost immediately. Five or six actors in patched long-johns postured and declaimed romantic sentiments in purple prose to another actor who sat cross-legged in the centre of the playing area chewing his nails. The playing area was covered with a large square of orange plastic. If this was not meant to be funny it should have been – the contrast between the sentiments and the setting was ludicrous enough, and the language was ridiculously florid. The rest of the audience, petrified by James's warnings to us and by Brecht's reputation, was rigidly silent. Annie was not so easily intimidated, and she laughed. Not loudly, not rumbustiously, quietly to herself, less audibly than if she had hiccupped or coughed, probably less noisily than an asthmatic breathing. Chris and I had been sufficiently overborne by James's strictures to try to hush her, which was appalling. Her laughter was an entirely appropriate reaction to what was happening in front of us. I think I would have reacted the same way if I had been alone.

We did not get a chance to see what came next, because in five minutes we were thrown out. First the woman who had sold us tickets came and offered to look after 'the little boy' while we watched the play. When we declined her offer, James ordered us to leave. James, Chris, and I had a preliminary shouting match outside the door, and then I sent Chris down the stairs with Annie so that I could tell James the full import of what he had done. At this stage James ordered us all to leave and threatened to call the police. I tried to explain Annie's situation to him, and at one point I even thought I was getting through. Then the shutters came down again. All that mattered to James was the play, 'a carefully orchestrated pattern of sound and silence', and he was completely unable to accept that Annie's reactions were those of a sentient being.

The next day I gave Annie the alphabet board and told her to say what she felt. She spelt, 'Why would James treat three patrons like that when he has so few?' and, 'You told James off properly.' I raised a question that had been bothering me. How would she like us to act in situations like that? I gave her the choice of 'quieter', 'as we were', and 'noisier'. She hovered between the last two and eventually came down on 'as we were': good manners came in there, probably. She then spelt 'I enjoy a fight, win or lose. People must be taught that we have rights.'

The theatre incident brought home to us a common problem for handicapped people. The normal world expects higher standards from handicapped people than it does from normal people. However embarrassed and upset the audience and the actors may have been by what was done to Annie, no one defended her. It was only later that we learnt that at a performance a few days earlier a drunken member of the audience had booed, laughed, catcalled and jeered throughout the play. No effort had been made to eject him, although his behaviour could have been described as ill-mannered, inappropriate, and prejudicial to the appreciation of the play by the rest of the audience. The noise Annie had been making was much softer than the noise made by members of the audience who had colds. Because she was handicapped her behaviour had to measure up to a standard which would be impossible for many normal people.

The first weekend out Annie had been relaxed with all the people she met. But the contact and the responses were at baby level, and no great effort was called for or expected on either side.

Anne's relationships developed along with her communication. The Joneses next door were typical. Sue was disconcerted by the extent of Annie's handicaps when she met her first but was able to adjust her reactions as Annie progressed. Her children, Sally and Jodie, on the other hand, had accepted Annie more easily at first, but were unable to comprehend the invisible changes which meant that they had to treat her as a teenager and not as a baby.

As time went on, however, Anne became much stiffer when meeting new people. She expected strangers to treat her as intelligent, and as far as she was concerned they were on trial until they proved themselves able to accept her ability. For this reason she always felt obliged to demonstrate her skills to any new acquaintance, and she would not relax until she had spelt something on the board and gauged the reaction. For a long time she was hypersensitive to any suggestion of being treated like a baby, and a friend of ours with a cheery motherly way of talking was often unnerved by seeing Annie dissolve in tears as she said no more than 'Hello' or 'Goodbye'. When out in public with complete strangers Annie was composed. No public slight ever reduced her to tears at the time, whatever it did to her later when she was alone with us. The strain was there, inevitably, but so was Annie's *savoir faire*.

When Annie started coming home regularly she needed to get some clothes of her own. Until then all her clothing had come from the institutional pool, and although I had tried to pick out items in good repair for her, they were still very dreary. Government institutions tend to order clothing in bulk, directly from the manufacturers, and this often means that special production lines are set up to make clothes that are unsaleable elsewhere. I could usually find Annie some clothes which fitted her, did not clash, and had not been hopelessly beaten out of shape by the laundry, but they still were not hers: somebody else had worn them last week and somebody else would wear them next week. Annie had not chosen them, and they added significantly to her 'oddness'. Handicapped people are already different from the rest of us. They do not need to have their differences highlighted by extraordinary clothing.

Annie needed the self-confidence that comes from knowing she was appropriately dressed. Her clothes had to communicate for her: 'I'm not dull, not dreary, not a baby; I do know what's what, and I have got a personality.' It was a tall order, and certainly not achievable in St Nicholas clothes.

One weekend we took Annie to Georges, a smart Melbourne department store, to buy her some really good clothes. Because of the discrepancy between her size and age, Annie did not have much choice about where she shopped. If she wanted to get the same kinds of clothes that those her age wore, she had to go to expensive children's shops.

She chose the clothes herself. I asked her if she would like a particular category of clothing such as slacks and if she said yes I would ask for all the variations in her size and offer them to her for approval. The shop assistants managed very well. We left Georges with a very trim, blue-grey, peasant-weave suit with red lining, and tops and tights and shoes to match. Annie had excellent taste. She liked strong, clear colours and could wear them successfully. She always knew what she wanted, and she never chose a garment that was not appropriate for her age. All the things she chose co-ordinated well.

From then on Annie and I shopped for clothes regularly, and she always made the final choice. I learnt quickly that it was pointless to do it any other way. Once I pressured her into accepting a white shirt that was reduced in price. She only wore it a couple of times before she grew out of it with relief and presented it to her friend Sasha, spelling out 'Give Sasha dye too.'

I was often lax about letting Annie choose what she wanted to wear each day. It was so much easier for me to pick them. Once when I had taken her out dressed very snappily, I thought, in a black skivvy and black velvet slacks she told me, 'It gives my ego hard knocks when you choose my clothes.' It was not that she disliked what I had chosen but it had not been her choice, and the clothes did not fit her mood.

To encourage Annie's spirit of independence Chris and I decided that she should have some pocket money. She was receiving the invalid pension, but it was paid to St Nicholas, and the hospital banked it and spent it without consulting her. Annie did not do badly. A colour television set and a page-turner were bought from it, but for everyday purposes she had nothing, no money in her purse to spend as she wished. She would be getting the pocket money from us, it is true, but the money would be hers to spend however she wanted.

We started giving her pocket money late in 1977. Her first purchase was a second-hand copy of *The Medium is the Massage*. She spent most of her money, however, on Christmas presents. In 1978 she saved up to buy a good radio and cassette player to replace the small transistor which I had given her years ago, and for the first time Annie had the experience of saving for something she wanted, instead of getting it immediately or going without. It meant that she had to learn to weigh up her priorities.

Annie had amazed us by the amount of general knowledge she had acquired from watching television. Once we realized the level she was at and the areas she was interested in, it was possible to channel her radio listening and television viewing constructively. There were difficulties when she was in St Nicholas because she had to go to bed early, but when she was at home we made sure that she did not miss out on worthwhile programmes. There were some particularly good radio programmes on the Australian Broadcasting Commission on Saturday afternoons which Annie enjoyed. On week days there were some excellent educational television programmes, and I used them as lessons. When Annie got her own television set she could still only watch it in the early evening, and she did not get a chance to say what she wanted to watch unless I was there. When I was not around or vigilant her set would be switched back to the channels that the nurses preferred, but television had certainly helped Annie to broaden her horizons.

In between the evening television shows I would read books to the children, a chapter or two a night. In this way we went through a lot of the classics, *Peter Pan*, *Alice in Wonderland*, *Treasure Island*, *Milly-Molly-Mandy*, and *The Magic Pudding*. Chris pointed out that these were much too young for Annie, but I argued that adults still enjoyed them and I thought they should be part of the background of any child brought up in an English-speaking country. Once the page-turner arrived Annie was able to be much more independent in her reading.

In July 1977 we took her to see her first film, *Nasty Habits*, which was about Watergate-type antics in a nunnery. After this we took her to films quite frequently. I was particularly keen for her to see some Australian films because I thought she needed background on the society she would have to live in. But even film going had its hazards for someone as sensitive as Annie. Slurs could come from the screen as well as from patrons and staff. Chris took Annie to see Woody Allen's comedy, *Annie Hall*. Everything went well until the scene in a bookshop when Woody says to Diane Keaton words to this effect: 'There are two kinds of lives, the horrible and the miserable. Being blind or crippled, that's horrible, I don't know how people like that can live. The rest of us are just miserable.' Annie began to protest in utterances of steadily rising pitch and volume until Chris took her out.

We took Annie to many of Melbourne's special places: the Royal Botanic Gardens, a bayside beach near the city, Acland Street, famous for its rich cakes and European style, and the Luna Park fun fair, where Annie revelled in the wild movement of the Whip and the Scenic Railway.

Annie's most ambitious and exciting trip that year was an excursion to Canberra, the national capital. Senior staff at St Nicholas were surprised that I wanted to take her, but nobody made any objections. When I asked her parents for their permission, they gave it happily.

We set off on Thursday 18 August. As Canberra is about 600 kilometres from Melbourne we had to fly, and it was

Annie's first flight. Despite the long journey and the stress of staying in a strange house with people she had never met, Annie was marvellously relaxed and took the first chance she was given to get at the alphabet board and show her skills.

It was the first time we had taken Annie out for a reasonable period (a whole four days) and for the first time in her life she was able to communicate a couple of sentences each day. She participated in a lively way in every conversation and often called the tune. As I was getting her ready for bed on Thursday night I noticed that her toe turned up as soon as her shoe was taken off. I tickled her feet trying to elicit a Babinsky reflex. When the others asked what I was doing I explained. Annie jumped up and down to show she wanted to contribute, and spelt out 'Badinisky [*sic*] reflex not present.' I imitated a standard test for the Moro reflex by knocking the back of the pusher beside her head, and asked her if she remembered being tested in this way. She spelt 'I have no Moro.' I had not mentioned the name of the reflex.

On Friday we went to some of Canberra's traditional tourist highlights. We began with the Australian War Memorial, which is an enormous military museum. I lifted Annie up to see the displays: a gas mask for a dog, trench signs made out of hammered bully-beef tins, dioramas of Gallipoli and Flanders, and I talked to her about the waste and suffering of war.

After lunch we went to Parliament House, where the Senate was having a special sitting. Senator Jean Melzer met us and took us around the Senate offices, and we signed the visitors' book. We watched about an hour of the debate from the President's Gallery.

It was a warm winter's day, and we strolled from Parliament House to the university. It had been a full day, and a taxing one.

On Saturday we had intended to go for a picnic in the country, but it rained and we had to settle for the university grounds. When Annie used the alphabet board her hand control was poor: her arm kept cramping, and her forearm bent right back across her face. I later learnt to identify this as a sign of tiredness, tension, or approaching illness. When we went home I put her to bed early, but she was miserable and later vomited.

By Monday she was quite chirpy again and ready to fight her own battles. During lunch with John Hannoush we were talking about Annie's mathematics. John was a mathematician, knew David Brownridge, and wanted to know what David and Annie were doing. I tried to explain, and I soon got into a tangle about their work. Annie spelt, 'David finished symbolic logic first,' but it was not enough to settle the argument. I was on the defensive because I was out of my depth, but Annie went on to the attack. She answered a couple of John's questions satisfactorily, and got her own back by making a rude pun on his name. It seemed that differences in terminology had caused the problem. David said he called Annie's work truth theory; John did not.

It had been a really successful trip, despite Annie's sickness, and it had shown that her handicaps were not an insurmountable barrier to travel. She had done all the traditional things a tourist does and being a teacher I followed up the trip with lessons on the founding of Canberra, parliamentary protocol and the Australian system of government. We flew back to Melbourne during the day so we were able to see the mountains and the snow. For Annie it was straight back to St Nicholas from the airport.

Christmas was approaching and although it was not ignored at St Nicholas, it was certainly not celebrated there in the same way as in people's homes. The wards would be decorated, toys would appear, mainly provided from a newspaper toy appeal, but the children were not given individual presents. There were certainly no stockings or Christmas cakes or any of the other delights of Christmas.

I remember one Christmas at St Nicholas finding a whole ward of children lying on mattresses in the playroom without an adult in sight and with nothing to amuse them: no television, no radio, no records.

On Christmas Eve in 1977, we brought Annie home for Christmas. On Christmas morning she opened her stocking, her first for fourteen years. It was mainly full of food, but there was also a ring, a ceramic mouse, some tights, and some bathers. We ate chocolates and I read to Annie until breakfast.

Chris's sisters came around for lunch and we exchanged presents around the tree. I took a photograph of Annie in her pusher in front of the tree with the presents piled around it, and the pile is higher than Annie.

Annie had chosen presents for us and bought them with her pocket money. She had spelt out with me what she wanted to give Chris: 'book, sci-fi, Asimov', and Chris had worked out a clever way of having her pick my present without my knowing what it was. He had telephoned St Nicholas the week before Christmas and asked me to bring Annie to the phone. I held the receiver to her ear while he gave her a list of choices, and then he asked me to ask her whether she wanted (1), (2), or (3). She chose (3), which on Christmas day turned out to be a bottle of French claret. Annie was given some marvellous presents: a poster book, a set of Chinese paper cut outs, Lorenz's book *On Aggression*, a necklace, *Catch-22*, Kate Greenway stickers, a beach towel, a carved wooden box to put them all in, and a touchlight. A touchlight is a bedside lamp with a metal base, which turns on and off with a touch of the hand anywhere on the base. Annie would be able to operate it. It pleased her enormously, and she operated it well.

When Annie had recovered from the effect of receiving so many presents, she spelt: 'Thanks to all, especially you.'

Annie's birthday on January 11 1978 fell in the middle of the week, and we held off celebrating it until the weekend. We collected Annie straight after lunch on Saturday and went to a puppet theatre to see *Alice in Wonderland*. Most of the audience were children and Annie managed the inevitable barrage of stares very well. On Sunday, before the guests started to arrive for her birthday lunch, she spelt out 'Thank everybody for their pres.' When I told her off for being too expectant, she finished by spelling, 'ence'. The first to arrive was Margaret, a friend of ours who had not met Annie before but had heard a lot about her. She had brought Annie Aldous Huxley's *Brave New World*. She handed it over and Annie *said*, 'Thank you.' Margaret replied, 'That's all right, don't mention it.' Margaret knew that Annie had communication problems, but Chris had not bothered to tell her that as far as we knew she had no intelligible speech. As far as Margaret was concerned, Annie was responding normally to a normal situation. Annie's words had been quite clear and unmistakable. Presumably she had thought the words and they had slipped through unscrambled. It has happened a handful of times since.

In the three weeks from Christmas until her birthday Annie spent twelve days out of the hospital. We went to two shows, the art gallery, the country, and swimming. Eight months after coming home with me for the first time, it was possible for her to do many of the same things when she was outside the hospital that a normal seventeen-year-old does. Even the presents she was given show how people's responses to her had changed since that first weekend when, thinking of her as a severely retarded girl, I had bought her a doll and a Little Golden Book.

She had come a long way.

ANNIE: Speech takes a lot of co-ordination, speaking at will, that is. Sometimes I say something without consciously trying, and it comes out more clearly than if I had tried hard. If I could speak without thinking I could talk clearly.

CHAPTER FIFTEEN

Back at St Nicholas I had been told that I was to work only with those children I was already teaching to spell. I had just added some young children to the group so this directive meant I was working with thirteen children. Whatever the hospital's motives for cutting back my sphere of activity, and however hard this was on the children I had been ordered to drop, it did mean that I had more time to spend with the Beanbaggers, and they could spend more time working together. At the same time they were all moved into one ward, and their sense of group identity undoubtedly increased. Children who had only been seeing one another for one or two afternoons a week and who had not much chance to explore each other's methods of communication were now together twenty-four hours a day. Their cots were together in one part of the ward, and there was at least the possibility of smiling at each other.

At this stage my rewards as a teacher were coming more from the other children than from Annie. Annie's literacy skills had advanced as far as I could take them, and any further improvement would be her own work. Her mathematics were already far beyond my understanding. David Brownridge, unfortunately, was not able to come as often as he had, and her education in this area unavoidably slackened. I could go on teaching her in specific areas – we began on French early in 1978 – but most of my efforts were devoted to the other children, and Annie was left to educate herself using the page-turner and her television set.

Now all the children in the group were spelling out free sentences. What they spelt was often more a cause for depression than for joy. I quoted samples of their work in reports I prepared for the authorities at the start of the new year. Mark the doormouse: 'I hate St Nicholas, so I sleep as much as possible.' Stephen: 'I am not retarded.' Phillip: 'I was undamaged at birth.' Sharon: 'I am handicapped, not stupid.' (That sentence struck me so forcibly that I had it made into a button for the children to wear when they went outside the hospital.) Shirley: 'It is kissing I miss most.' Noelene: 'Why are we retarded?' As usual, there was no response to the claim that the children could communicate, or to what they said.

Annie's relationships with the other children fluctuated. They were indubitably her friends, but she became extremely jealous if I gave any of them the attention she felt should be hers. It came out especially in relation to feeding. The strength of her reaction when she saw me feeding another child became increasingly irrational. At first she grizzled when I fed anybody else, later she yelled, and by the time we went out to the Dandenong Ranges with the whole group for the 1977 Christmas party she screamed uncontrollably.

Annie knew she was wrecking the day for herself, but she could not help it. She yelled and screamed so much at lunch that she had to be parked away in a corner of the garden. Some of the other children were difficult to feed, and the volunteers who had come to help were not used to them. I had to feed them and Annie just had to accept Chris feeding her or wait.

It was a very gruelling time for both of us. I suppose she wanted reassurance that she was my first concern. It was understandable, but I was very glad when she got over it.

I liked the way it happened, She did it for Stephen. He is a red-headed boy with a fetching smile and a tendency to be easily discouraged. First thing in the new year Annie spelt out 'Tonight feed Stephen.'

'Why?', I asked. It was something of an about-face.

'Stephen is too thin,' she spelt.

She knew I was worried about him, but as usual Annie did not tell me immediately what was really worrying her.

The next day she spelt out, 'Feed Stephen tonight.' I told her that I would be trying to feed Stephen every night. 'Why do you feel you have to say it again?', I asked.

'A doctor said Stephen is too thin to live for long if he doesn't gain weight,' Annie replied. She was upset, partly I suspect because she felt that she had contributed to Stephen's condition, and that I would have fed him earlier if she had not been so difficult about it.

I had been feeding Annie her lunch and dinner since November. Now I added Stephen and fed them together. From the time I began to feed Stephen it was obvious that he had a problem. He vomited at almost every meal. When I reported it and tried to get a doctor to see him, it took some time to get through the system. I had to spend quite a lot of time with Stephen, because getting anything to stay down meant feeding him very slowly, with numerous pauses. If it did not stay down it meant that I had to mop up and start again, and it often took me an hour or an hour and a half. Stephen was finally examined by a doctor and a haemoglobin test done two weeks after I had reported his condition. His haemoglobin was 6.2, half his normal level, and he had started to vomit 'coffee-grounds', usually the sign of a bleeding ulcer. As soon as it was discovered that he was ill, I was forbidden to feed him. Stephen was not consulted. Several more days passed before any action was taken on the haemoglobin reading. St Nicholas is called a hospital, but doctors did not visit the wards every day, and the sister did not feel that Stephen's symptoms justified asking one to make a special trip. When a doctor came she was so stunned by the haemoglobin count that she called in a paediatrician who suggested that Stephen was suffering from anorexia nervosa, a psychological complaint involving a pathological unwillingness to eat! and told me that I was not to feed Stephen unless ordered to do so, as his welfare was the responsibility of the ward. In the end Stephen was transferred to Ward 3, the only ward in the hospital where there was a trained sister who could administer the iron injections that had been prescribed for him. The original idea was that Stephen would come back to Ward 2 to join the others when his course of iron injections was over. He even got a clearance from the paediatrician. As usual, however, politics prevailed. I was in disgrace for various misdemeanours which had nothing to do with Stephen, and Stephen was made the scapegoat. It was ruled that he should stay in Ward 3 away from all his friends and all the children he could communicate with, and he has been there ever since. He was able to join the other children for lessons for five hours a day but on weekends he was completely isolated.

Stephen does not have Annie's steely determination. In March he spelt out to me 'Request power to be given to Justice of the Peace to take my life.' It was Stephen, also, who spelt out 'Has God ignored us?'

I made an appointment to see Dr Barlow, the Director of Mental Retardation Services, to discuss Stephen. He was most sympathetic, and I felt he believed me. He was rather at a loss about what to do, but he said he would approach the St Nicholas authorities. As usual, nothing came of this. Stephen's situation remained completely unchanged, and I was given one of my regular blastings for not going through the 'normal channels'.

Chris and I had talked it over and decided that if nobody else was going to do anything to help Stephen we would have to. The obvious thing was to start to bring him home for weekends. Ironically, I had no trouble in getting permission. He could go out for weekends with me but he was too 'ill' or 'frail' to join his friends in another ward of the hospital.

Not surprisingly, this was a very stressful period for Annie. She had started it all off by asking me to feed Stephen, and now there was no way to stop the process that was leading to her having to share us at home as well as at St Nicholas. On top of that Annie had less time to be taught by me and less time to communicate with me, particularly at any length.

On 18 March 1978 we took her out to visit the Old Melbourne Gaol and Museum. When we returned to St Nicholas I was sufficiently worried to use the alphabet board, despite the fact that it was 6.20 p.m. and Chris's family was coming to dinner at 7.

My diary entry gives a fair idea of the kinds of problems we were having.

We started well, though slowly, but I tired quickly and was very conscious of the time and got crabby when things started to get confused. Annie's arm seemed to be tight. However every time I got mad she was suddenly able to move it perfectly well for the next few letters, before going back to the bottom left corner where she would point very clearly to four or five letters in a row, but say 'no' to each of them when asked. Recently our rapport on communication seems to have disappeared and it all seems very slow and difficult. Part of this is probably because I'm tired and tense; but part is certainly due to the fact that Annie's face isn't providing the amount of feed-back it used to. Her old yes/no at the board (squeeze tongue - yes, tongue unmoved - no) seems to have disappeared and to get a clear yes/no takes ages. Her eyes are also not as expressive as they were. It's as though she is shutting me out, applying a protective coating perhaps. I feel that there are two obvious explanations for the problems that Annie and I have been having over the last few weeks. (1) She doesn't like me.

(2) She is afraid that I don't like/am rejecting her. I spoke about these possibilities to Annie saying that if it was (1) I was sorry but she would have to tolerate me until she was independent on Possum, and that it certainly wasn't (2). I said that the closest relationships weren't always sunshine and roses and that e.g. Chris and I often had periods of coolness lasting some time and not to worry about resenting me, or whatever, that it was normal. I got a sympathetic response when I said that it was a difficult time for both of us and that I doubted if either of us was sleeping well, and that this would obviously exacerbate things. I explained that I generally get angrier with people that I'm close to than not, because I have high expectations of them. Finished this in ward while changing Annie. Kissed her goodnight particularly affectionately. Radio on. Goodnighted others. It sounded suspiciously as if Annie was trying not to cry as I left her chatting with the night nurse for a minute or two. Visited Stephen briefly.

Calm and controlled personal relationships are not my forte. I don't like the responsiblity inherent in close ties which is the main reason I don't want to have children. I really like and admire Annie, and I don't see our association as just being a temporary one, however at the moment my relationship with her and with all the Beanbaggers is being poisoned by a 'why me' feeling on my part (which I feel I am being most unsuccessful in concealing) brought about by my knowledge that they are a responsibility which I can't (and in most ways don't want to) shed, and which seems to daily increase in weight, with no end in sight. Sisyphus and I have a lot of gripes in common!

On Monday Annie spelt, partly on the Possum, 'To love was having difficulties I didn't see. Tell Chris I love him too.' As far as I know it was her first explicit emotional commitment.

Fortunately for Stephen Ward 3 was having staff problems and soon I was ordered to feed him. This made life more difficult for Annie. There was no time now for the leisurely meals that we had been having since Stephen had been transferred. I had to feed Annie as quickly as possible to have time to dash over to Ward 3. The Possum also played its part in increasing the pressure. We were all suffering from frustration and disappointed hopes. At least by this time I had managed to be allowed to do evening work again, which helped a bit.

Easter came early in 1978 and provided an excellent opportunity to get us on an even keel again. Annie went on a picnic and had her first taste of peanut butter sandwiches. More significantly, she had her first experience of being alone. On Saturday morning Chris had dashed off to the market. I was getting ready to go to the shop for supplies to tide us over the holidays when it started to rain. I had no wet weather clothes for Annie. I had to leave her at home. I was rather dubious about it, but the alternative seemed to be a shortage of food over Easter and I was sure that Annie would feel the hardship as keenly as any of us. She said she did not mind. I put her on a blanket on the floor in the living-room with a radio to listen to, and I shut the dog outside. She could not injure herself accidentally, and barring fire or flood she was fine. It is obviously undesirable for anyone who is helpless to be left alone for any length of time, but I think it is probably a good idea for all handicapped people to learn to deal with limited 'desertions'. It is bound to happen occasionally.

After lunch Annie asked us to take her to church and we arranged for her to go to an Anglican midnight mass.

On Sunday we ate enormous quantities of chocolate Easter eggs and went to a fifties revival show at the scene of our debacle last year, the alternative theatre in Carlton. The ambience was very different this time, we had no problems, and Annie did not seem at all bothered by past associations. She was in fits of laughter throughout and so, this time, was everybody else. Annie woke up in the middle of the night and was crying. I gave her a drink, but I think she wanted the contact. I think she was sorry about the holiday ending.

On 5 April the boy in the cot next to Stephen's died in

the night. On 11 April a girl in Stephen's ward died. Her death was particularly harrowing. She died slowly over some weeks, in considerable pain, near the entrance to the ward in full view of the children and staff. Anybody who watched television had to watch her dying. Meal time after meal time I fed Stephen only metres from her oxygen tent, leaping up every few minutes when her breathing missed a beat to check that she was still alive.

She was not able to swallow, and as St Nicholas had no facilities for intravenous feeding she became dehydrated, but she was still expected to produce a daily bowel movement, and when she failed to produce it the standard remedies were applied. First she was given a pill, and then a suppository. When an enema was suggested, the ward staff rebelled. They were threatened with dismissal, and the enema was administered by the nurse in charge of the ward.

The nurses at St Nicholas have a superstition that deaths go in threes, and after any two deaths in close sequence there is a lot of speculation about who is going to be the third. I should not have been surprised when Stephen spelt out on 12 April, 'I'm goddamn dying.' He had overheard the nurses. He was aware of the irony. Less than a month before he had asked to be killed and now he was complaining about dying. But now he had something to hope for. I had told him that Chris and I would be taking him home at weekends as soon as the formalities were completed.

April 14 marked the anniversary of Annie's first visit to our house and everybody she had met then made a special point of coming around to visit. On Saturday we listened to a radio programme which brought us face to face with an issue we had not talked about before. It was a programme on the economics of health care. What value do we place on a life? Is there an expenditure beyond which we should not go to preserve life? If so, what is it? Annie spelt out, 'As I take a lot should I die?' I replied that the cost of keeping her alive should be a community cost, not a health cost. The cost of her care, then about $10 000 a year at St Nicholas, was no greater than that of most children. Sally and Jodie next door, for instance, were taking their mother out of the work-force, absorbing a slab of their father's earnings, and they were using educational facilities that Annie had no access to. I am not sure if it was the kind of answer Annie wanted. She may have been asking us to think what our opposition to preserving life at all costs implied.

On Sunday we ran into communication troubles again. Anne's communication was usually at her own wish. She would jump up and down to show that she wanted to spell something, I would check with her yes/no responses, and then I would get the board and she would take it from there, spelling of her own free will and not in answer to any question or suggestion.

Aileen and John and Damian and Bill came, bringing cards and food for afternoon tea, so that when I asked Annie if she wanted to say something she may have thought I was ordering her. Bill, who is six, kept saying, 'What will she spell? Will she spell, "I am Annie?"' and both of the boys kept guessing letters and words rather disconcertingly. When she got as far as 'I am Ann' Annie gave up.

After everybody had left we had another go and extended it to 'I am annually given' before she jammed up again. The trouble with Annie's jamming up is that not only do her arm movements become awkward but her yes/no responses fall apart, and it becomes impossible to continue. It gets worse if she is tired, and it also tends to happen if she has not got anything particular she wants to say and feels that she is 'performing'. It also happens if I am tired or cross, and then I am less tolerant than usual. On this occasion I was really upset that Annie's anniversary weekend was ending like this, and I showed it. After we had both had a quarter of an hour to relax I asked here if she would like to try to finish the sentence, and I think she was quite relieved to be able to redeem herself. Quickly she spelt, 'Such a good time that I can't wait until next year.'

St Nicholas was finding its way into the headlines again. The Fire Brigade had labelled the place a fire risk, and the teachers had gone to the press about the complete lack of any suitable teaching facilities. The Health Commission reacted in the least appropriate way. It was announced that St Nicholas would be given an enormously expensive new sprinkler system – money that would have been much better spent housing the children elsewhere – and children were packaged off to any other institution in the state that had vacancies. Often the results were tragically inappropriate. Two deaf and blind children from St Nicholas were sent to an institution at Colac in the country which had no other such children, no programmes for deaf and blind children, and no staff who had worked with deaf and blind children. St Nicholas was not well equipped for them, but we did have some help from teachers from Monnington in setting up their programmes. I spent a lot of time trying to explain to reporters why the wholesale shipping-out of children was not appropriate and I spent a lot of time trying to ensure that none of the children in the group was on the list to go. I had been told that they would not be separated, and I was reassured by this until at the beginning of May I found one of the nurses packing a suitcase for Noelene. The Director of Nursing said she was to be sent to Colac the next day. After a frantic twenty-four hours in which I decided that the only way to stop the transfer would be to make the whole thing public, her name was taken off the list, and we all relaxed. Noelene spelt, 'I'm happy I'm not going away.'

I was trying to teach the children about people with other handicaps and how they coped with them. We talked about Helen Keller, about Braille, and about a deaf and blind girl in Melbourne. We had a visit from Kaye Gooch, now one of Annie's dearest friends, herself a spastic who is legally blind, deaf and has a speech disability. She was a tremendous inspiration: she holds down a completely normal job in the Taxation Department despite three handicaps, any one of which would entitle her to an invalid pension.

I saw the State College videotape for the first time and found it most encouraging. It was generally agreed that it would convince any but the most hardened unbeliever. Several hundred students had seen the tape by the end of that year, and from what I heard they had no doubt about the validity of Annie's communication. Several students recognized me later at functions and surprised me by saying that viewing the tape was the most memorable part of their whole course and the thing that had meant most to them.

On Monday 3 July 1978 the world turned upside down. I collected Stephen from Ward 3 and we went over to Ward 2 to find the children on the verandah as usual watching *Sesame Street*. Dennis had died in his beanbag. I tried to give him mouth-to-mouth resuscitation and heart massage but he did not breathe again. As I worked on him I thought I must be dreaming: I thought things did not happen this way; soon I would wake up and he would be all right. It was a terrible way to die, and horrible for the other children who had to watch my attempt to save him.

When the Superintendent came and it was clear that Dennis was not going to revive, I started to cry. Later on I was told that this was unprofessional behaviour: one should not cry when a child dies. Dennis had lived thirteen years in St Nicholas. If I didn't cry for him, who would? But I did not cry for long. I had to pull myself together and go out and see the children to tell them that Dennis was dead. Annie was crying quietly, so was Noelene; she had been Dennis's favourite. Lesley was crying, but then she cried a lot anyway. The others all looked sad and subdued. The nurses thought this showed that they must be constipated, and they wanted to give them all suppositories. At least I managed to stop that.

Sharon was moved into the vacant beanbag quite literally before it was cold. I took her out of it, and carried the beanbag upstairs to the physiotherapy section where nobody would know about its past. I moved Dennis's cot out of the group's area of the ward and gave his toys to a child in another ward.

Dennis was my favourite in the group, almost more than Annie. He was appallingly handicapped, even compared to the other children. It was impossible for him to lie straight or to lie on his back, because he was so spastic that his head would push right back. That may have killed him. He had gone blue a few weeks before, and when I questioned him about it later he said that it was because he had been incorrectly positioned. He had almost suffocated in a beanbag once when he was with me, and I had spoken to the nurses on the ward, showing them the right way to position him. As it happened there were a number of new staff on the ward the day he died.

I was fond of Dennis because he was so gutsy, and he had a terrific sense of humour. He had more difficulty using the alphabet board than anyone else in the group, but he persevered regardless. Occasionally it was possible to pick up a few words of his speech. Once when I had been trying to get him to point out the answer to a sum on the board and he had been just making noises, a volunteer working at the other end of the room called out, 'Is the answer five? That's what he's been saying.' It was.

Because his head was pushed so far back he was very difficult to feed, and for some reason nursing staff seemed to feel that it was easier to feed him if you mixed his main course with his pudding. It was a common practice in the hospital, but Dennis hated it and complained to me with increasing virulence about it: 'Up the nurses. Give mine a taste of mixture.' He was anxious for an independent means of communication, and when word came that the Possum was being delivered he spelt out with a wry smile, 'I hate a fuss. First go Possum mine.' One of the last things he spelt was 'Is our house possible? Who pays?' We had been talking about the possibility of the children in my group living together in a half-way house outside St Nicholas when I put in my submission to the Schools Commission. As it happened it was Dennis who paid.

On the afternoon of Dennis's death the consultant paediatrician came round to assess the intelligence of some of the children. It took him from 2.30 p.m. to 3.15 p.m., three-quarters of an hour for five children, including Annie. All were assessed lying flat on their backs and I was not asked to help. He did not want to know their yes/no responses, he said, that might bias his assessment.

Some days afterwards Annie and Stephen came home and Annie spelt, 'Dennis was crying out "help" but I ignored him.'

'Why?', I asked.

'He . . . it went quiet immediately,' she replied.

'Did you realize what happened?,' I asked.

'No. I thought he was okay. No one else heard.'

'Are you sure of that?'

'Yes.'

Angela, the baby of the group, had the last word: 'Is our house possible?'

'Yes,' I replied.

'Shame Dennis didn't live to see it,' she spelt.

Two weeks after Dennis's death I came in one morning to find Stephen in an oxygen tent. His breathing had become distressed during breakfast and the nurses had whisked him into the oxygen tent straight away. He was only semi-conscious when I saw him, but his colour was starting to come back. The doctors came in later, diagnosed bronchopneumonia, and put him on penicillin. By the afternoon he was livelier, and I was able to give him a drink. The worst thing about being sick in St Nicholas, I think, must be being nursed as an inanimate object with no right to be told anything and no right to have any feelings – never asked, 'Do you feel thirsty? Do you have a headache?' It must have been terrifying for Stephen to be bundled into the oxygen tent like that. Nobody made any attempt to explain that going into the tent does not necessarily mean you are at death's door. And of course everybody was discussing his chances of survival in front of him on the assumption that he could not understand a word.

I took Annie upstairs and told her about it, but I did not tell the other children.

The next morning Leonie was upset. When I asked her why she spelt out, 'Annie said Steve in okcigen tent.' I asked her what Annie had said Stephen had. Leonie spelt out, 'Noomonia.' I was stunned. It meant that the children could communicate with each other. I had wondered about this before because there was a fair bit of vocalization by the children, but I had never really taken it as a serious possibility. Stephen was out of the tent and fully conscious by this time, and I was able to reassure Leonie about him. After that I went and ticked off Annie for passing on confidences. She laughed and several of the others who had been listening gave each other knowing looks. I started to quiz the children about who understood whom. Phillip said he did not understand anybody and nobody understood him, which was a lie. Leonie said she did not understand Angela. The next day I took Annie over to see Stephen. I had to restore my credibility with the group after not having told them he was sick, and I thought she should see his recovery herself.

I did not follow up the issue of their language immediately. It took a while to sink in. But it was confirmed and rounded off a week later, when Annie complained to me privately about the lack of sex life in St Nicholas. The next day Phillip spelt out wickedly, 'I could help Annie with her problems.' The children were talking a lot more than they had been. Every time I left the room there was more conversation and laughter. It was not like anything I had heard from them before. Now the secret of their language was out they did not have to be careful. From a distance it sounded just like normal teenagers chatting. Leonie would 'say' something and Lesley would crack up.

While feeding Annie dinner I thought over the implications. It affected all sorts of things. I had a quiet chat with Sharon, who had been worrying me because of her inattention during lessons, and I asked her why she kept laughing at the wrong times. Did the others say things to make her laugh? She said they did. I remember the trick from my own classroom days.

Mark said he could understand nine children, seven of them in the group. Stephen, Shirley, Phillip and young Angela were non-speakers.

'Who are the two children you mentioned who are not in the group?', I asked.

'JB and SK,' he replied.

'How bright do you think they are?'

'If rilising [realizing] St Nicholas is terrible means you are bright then they are.'

Annie was abnormally subdued the following weekend. She did not want to do anything or go anywhere or eat anything. When I took her back to St Nicholas in the evening she wanted to use the alphabet board and she spelt out very quickly, 'I'm hopping mad that we kept our speech a secret fearing that we wouldn't be believed.' That may have been the reason. I think part of it was wanting to keep something in reserve that I did not know about, just in case. It certainly demonstrated Annie's leadership over the others that she was able to get them to agree to keep it from me as long as they did. Possibly it explained why the other children's maths homework was consistently correct.

Stephen and Annie were still coming home together. As Annie was still reluctant to talk in front of us we thought it might help if we could tape her talking to Stephen, play it back, and analyse it. We set up a cassette recorder surreptitiously one night but Annie was abnormally quiet. She only really made any noise at about 9.30 in the morning, when I was still in bed. I played the tape through later in private and the main thing seemed to be Annie calling out 'Get up! Get up!' In the evening Annie spelt out 'Doubt if playing the tapes with Chris will help you understand me.' It is hopeless trying to conceal things from Annie. Her hearing is simply too good. I asked her if she had any comments or suggestions and she spelt, 'Play them and I'll tell you what I said.' I played her the morning's tape, saying that I thought I could pick out a couple of words. I asked her what she had been saying. She spelt, 'Get up' and we went through the tape phrase by phrase with her telling me what was said.

I had been aware of jealousies between the children but they emerged very clearly at a Christmas party which Jean Melzer attended. She was introduced to everyone and handed out presents. Annie got the *Penguin Book of English Verse* and, as an extra, a doll with McDonald tartan trews which Jean had got in Scotland. Mark spelt 'Thanks' on behalf of the group, and Annie, who had been peeved throughout, practically exploded. She wanted Jean to be her friend exclusively. I asked her if she had anything to say. She spelt 'Many thanks. Happy Hogmany.' Mark felt he had been slighted and burst into tears, and then Annie started to cry too.

At times I felt like the old woman who lived in a shoe. Annie was going through a desperate in-between stage: some of her friends were leaving Melbourne or splitting up, and the rest were having to be shared with the group or with Stephen. I could understand something of what she felt: do they like me because I am me, or are they just kind to me in the same way as they would be to all the children because we are so handicapped? The sad thing is that the people she was most worried about were devoted to her and had to bend over backwards when they were with the group to give an appearance of even-handedness, but she could not have known that and it was not the kind of problem that could be rectified simply by telling her. She had to see for herself that she could afford to share people, that they were not automatically going to walk out on her when they saw the others, and that you do not have to have someone's undivided attention all the time to feel confident of their affection for you.

ANNIE: We spoke a mixture of Yugoslav and English which we later called Yuggish. Communication took a long time because we had to repeat things. Subtle meanings were impossible. Watching each other was vital to understanding our speech; I could understand a lot from the other children's mime. We all used facial expressions to give emphasis.

Children who were admitted before they learnt to speak never heard English spoken by people without severe speech problems. When we first came to St Nicholas we could not understand any of the adults in the strange new world in which we found ourselves until we learnt Yugoslav. Because of this, speech became a secret that separated us from them. For a time no child understood an adult, and no adult understood a child. The children learnt; the adults did not. My speech has been understood by a number of children but never by any adult. We could understand everybody, but no one understood us.

Because the adults could not understand us they shut us up every time we tried to talk. Sometimes I was hit because I talked with other children, and the nurses thought I was screaming without reason. Since we were always with nurses, opportunities for speech were few. Speaking became harder when the nurses upset us because our vocal problems were exacerbated by tightness. Tightness is the major problem in cerebral palsy, and all the intelligent children had cerebral palsy. Some kids stopped talking altogether.

Until Rosemary Crossley came to St Nicholas we did not know there were ways for non-handicapped people to talk with us. Slowly stiff arms began to gesture to augment tongues. This made voices less important and meant that some kids who could not speak very much could still communicate. The method we used was that questions could be answered using hands. You asked a child if he had something to say, and if he gave the 'yes' sign you asked him questions until you got the subject, and then you asked more questions until you guessed correctly. Cursory questioning was all there was time for: it took ages for me to ask the questions because I spoke so slowly and had to repeat myself so often to be understood. This type of interview stopped when we were put to bed because the partitions made it impossible to use gestures.

I used to try to teach the others things. Once Rosie started teaching me to spell I tried to teach the others.

I did not tell Rosie about our speech because I thought she would not believe it. Normal people take it for granted that if you are incomprehensible to them then no one can understand you, and Rosie is the worst person I know at understanding handicapped speech.

Chapter Sixteen

I was worried about the implications of my work for the parents. Parents of children in St Nicholas were not encouraged to take an interest in the progress of their children. Once they had put them into the hospital they were encouraged not to worry about them, to put the whole episode behind them. The hospital did not want to be bothered by anxious parents.

Some parents were turned off by the hospital's attitude and stopped coming to see their child; some, including Annie's parents, would visit a few times a year; some maintained close contact, coming every week.

Plainly, it was going to be a delicate matter to help Annie's parents to accept her development. Almost the first instruction that the Superintendent gave me was that Annie's parents were not to be told about my work with her. He said later in a report:

I did have discussions with Ms Crossley about informing Anne's parents of her progress and I indicated that in my view the child had not been proven to have made enough progress in communication to warrant informing her parents. The reason for this was because I did not wish to raise any false hopes with the parents ... I did direct Ms Crossley not to inform Mr and Mrs McDonald of Anne's progress with communication.

The gap between what I knew about Annie and what her parents knew widened steadily. I thought that Mrs

McDonald trusted me, and I could see that she would feel I had betrayed her if she found out about Annie from somebody else; I knew I would be fired if she found out about her from me. It was not impossible that she would find out by accident. One day I came in and found a new doll hanging on Annie's cot. Her mother had taken her out to a fete in the suburb of Kew. I wondered what Mrs McDonald had made of the mathematics homework I had left on the bars of Annie's cot. When I asked Annie she spelt out, 'Left doll for you.' Her mother had left the doll in the nurses' office and she had not seen the work on the cot bars. The situation had been saved, but it would not be long before her parents sensed that something was happening.

When I rang Mrs McDonald in 1977 to ask for her permission to take Annie to Canberra I suggested that she should ask the hospital for a progress report. She came to Melbourne and saw one of the doctors at St Nicholas, but she was told almost nothing; she was told that I was saying that Annie was doing things that other people did not believe she was doing, but she was not told what they were, and she was not asked to have a look for herself.

When DEAL was formed one of the first issues it discussed was the need to inform the parents. The committee's suggestions went unheeded. In 1978 I wrote to the Superintendent a number of times asking that the parents be told, but my requests were rejected.

There were two sides to this. I was worried about the children's relationships with their parents. What do you do when you have been ordered not to allow a mother to communicate with her daughter? Lesley spelt out, 'I want to talk to Mum.' She was terribly frustrated by not being able to get through, and her mother, who came in almost every week and was very close to her, could feel this. She kept asking me what I thought was troubling Lesley, and I had to evade her question. I felt very badly about it.

Towards the end of 1978, about eighteen months after

I had begun my work with Annie, I finally got a chance to make contact with her parents on an appropriate level. We wanted to take Annie to Canberra again, and I rang Mrs McDonald to ask her permission. I still was not allowed to speak about Annie's abilities, but I did ask her mother if she had seen the videotape of Annie which had been made a year ago. It was the first she had heard of it. She asked me if things were being bought for Annie out of her pension. I told her about the page-turner. She was curious, and when she pressed me to explain I told her I was not allowed to discuss Annie's ability or the work we were doing together. I said she should ask the Superintendent for a report.

A month later she came down to Melbourne. What ensued was a classic example of the power of the status quo. I was told at 11 a.m. on 13 December 1978 that Mrs McDonald was at the hospital and that the Superintendent had said I could show her Annie's work. I took Annie upstairs where Mrs McDonald was waiting with Annie's sister Roslyn, aged 11, and a nursing sister. I suggested we all go into the playroom to see what Annie had been doing. Mrs McDonald wandered over to have a look at the page-turner, but I steered her away from it. I thought the book Annie was reading, a difficult mathematics text, would be too much for her to take at this stage. I began to set up the magnetic letters on the board. 'Oh, I don't believe this,' said Mrs McDonald. Annie was fairly relaxed. On the way up I had suggested to her that she keep her comments low key unless she had something special to say. She spelt out, 'Tell Dad television teaches you some things better than books.' Mrs McDonald and Roslyn began to laugh. Apparently there is a standing family argument about television, and Annie's father insists that it is ruining the morals and education of the young. I was very rigorous with the pointing, and the sentence took about half an hour to spell out. By the end Mrs McDonald was saying the letters first. She asked me how long Annie had been using the board, when the videotape had been made, and how I had taught Annie to spell. I went over the story quickly but in quite a lot of detail. I drew her a set of circles and showed her the blocks.

Mrs McDonald told me that after Annie was born she and her husband had been told Annie would never be able to do anything, and that this had been repeated by expert after expert.

We went back to Ward 2 and kept on talking as I fed Annie lunch. I asked Mrs McDonald, without probing too deeply, a bit about any physiotherapy Annie had been given as a child. She said that they had tried standing her in plaster casts when she was very young, but that Annie had become hysterical and it was stopped.

Mrs McDonald said the family was coming to the Chrismas party on Saturday to bring Annie a 'treat'. I wondered what it was and whether they would have second thoughts about giving it to her after what I had shown them today.

I thought then that we were over the top. I imagined we had come through the revelation smoothly and that when Mrs McDonald had thought about it for a while she would be able to establish a new relationship with Annie. I was wrong. I had underestimated the strength of the misconceptions that had been inculcated in Annie's parents by the events of the last eighteen years, and I had greatly overestimated the effect of seeing something yourself as against hearing a contrary assertion from a doctor. If there had been unanimity in St Nicholas about Annie we might have got through the transition without an upset. As it was, Mrs McDonald did not ask to see Annie spelling again.

In mid-1978 Dr Barlow resigned as Director of Mental Retardation Services. He celebrated his resignation with an article in the *Australian Medical Journal* explaining how important it was to do away with large institutions in favour of family group homes. DEAL made contact with Dr Rosemary West, the new Acting Director, as soon as it could. First impressions were very promising. She came to see Annie spell. She even brought the Superintendent of the hospital with her. Although Annie did no more than spell 'Thur' in answer to a question about what day it was, it was more than she had been able to spell out before to anyone in authority. Dr West also saw the State College videotape and seemed to find it convincing. DEAL continued the search for a house where the children could live together. We looked at Swinburne House, a residential centre in the suburb of Black Rock for children who could not live at home, and in September Dr West wrote a letter which said:

We would be interested in seeing Swinburne House set up to serve multiply physically handicapped children who appear to be functioning at a higher cognitive level but who need very intensive educational programmes so that their developmental gain can be assessed.

It was the most positive thing we had seen written about the children by anyone in authority. Unfortunately the project went no further than that.

Dr West had started well, but the rigidities of the bureaucracy made short work of good intentions. DEAL had a meeting with her at the beginning of December to discuss the children's early bed times. After the meeting she wrote to DEAL:

I have discussed the problem of the children retiring to bed so early with the appropriate person. There are major problems with regard to cleaning the wards and preparing for the next day . . . One can appreciate the need to put the children to bed early so that all these chores can be accomplished. I have been assured that the matter will be looked into. I must point out, however, that this problem is a very real one in large institutions, and St Nicholas is certainly not unique in this regard . . . I would be grateful if the matter could be allowed to rest at this point. We must allow the senior staff at St Nicholas to administrate the hospital in the manner, which, by experience, has proven to be the most efficient.

Efficiency seemed to be her entire justification for putting teenagers to bed at 4.30 p.m.

From mid-1978 onwards I thought constantly of going to the press. Every time I reached desperation point, however, another carrot would be dangled in front of my nose, something that would be lost to us if there were any publicity.

Dennis's death and Stephen's illness had increased my sense of desperation. It seemed that nobody who was in a position to do anything cared. I could not understand how people could know about the situation and ignore it. Everybody needs protection against bureaucratic bungling, but children need it more than most. If an injustice had been done then it should have been remedied immediately.

By this time we all seemed to have acquired fixed roles: the children as victims, me as agitator, the Health Commission as an unapproachable monolith. Despite saying fervently that I would stick with the fight until the children got out, deep down I was thinking that they never would. I went through the routine each day at St Nicholas, and I went through the motions of agitating outside, because there did not seem any alternative.

Chris Biddle, an occupational therapist who came from Yooralla in a voluntary capacity to help me with the children's communication problems, recommended that we use standing-frames. I had asked her to come to help us work on the Possum, but by the time she was given permission from the hospital the Possum was not working. Her view was that we had to start right back at first principles and get the children properly positioned and stabilized before we started work on their hand skills. She thought that as many children as possible should be stood regularly in standing-frames. Because we had no callipers, standing involved making plaster slabs moulded to the shape of the back of the leg and then bandaging them to the child at each session. It was a particularly time-consuming process. As we only had one standing-frame we could not stand the whole group at once. We had to bandage, stand, unbandage, bandage, stand, unbandage. In one way it was very good for Annie. She had always been reluctant to have anything to do with splinting and tight strapping, and her first reaction to these plasters was unfavourable. She gradually overcame her dislike, however, and was able to stand for progressively longer periods without complaint. On 10 October I wrote in my diary: 'Annie in plasters for two hours. Fine.'

Eventually both my back and my enthusiasm for plasters gave out. At Christmas, when the teachers were on holidays, I stopped using them. It was becoming clear that I had to develop a set of priorities. The children were so disabled in so many areas that I had to make choices. Rightly or wrongly, I decided to develop skills that would help the children to leave St Nicholas. Once they left St Nicholas it would be possible to catch up on the remedial work they needed in other areas. Physical ability was not going to take the children out of the hospital. For that they would need courage and their intellectual skills, shown, if possible, through independent communication. It would only be worth while going on with the plasters if there were a possibility that the Possum would be repaired. From then on I concentrated mainly on academic skills, although I did keep trying for an independent system of communication for the children.

Two practical problems faced me with machine communication: we needed a machine, and we needed suitable seating to give the children a chance to operate it. The first problem was the easier. I designed a machine myself, based on an article I had read in an American magazine, and I had it made up by an electrician. It was simple, cheap, and portable, being little more than a pointer that went around a dial until you pressed a switch to stop it or that stayed still until you pressed a switch to start it. The switch was light and simple to operate, and the dial had a metal front so that you could draw on it or stick pictures or magnetic letters to it. I wanted a machine that could be used by either children or adults: toddlers can use this one to choose between their toys, and adults with good physical control can use it to choose letters of the alphabet. I decided to call it the Wombat, and I had a number of them made. One of the ironies of the situation is that both Yooralla and the Spastic Society have bought some, and they are being used by children and adults as a major means of communication.

The Wombat worked well, and a talented voluntary helper made switch-holders to help the children work it, but the problem of seating remained. Mounting a switch in an optimum position for someone who is sitting in a beanbag is impossible: if he pushes the switch he changes position in the beanbag and he changes his orientation to the switch. Any kind of electronic equipment requires suitable chairs. Together with the physiotherapist and the head teacher at St Nicholas, I put in a submission to the Schools Commission for a grant to buy chairs. It was rejected. The Schools Commission grants for residential institutions were given to provide luxuries. It was thought that chairs were not a luxury and that the Health Commission should pay for them, but it refused. The children missed out again.

I had been emphasizing the need for seating more vociferously since Dennis died, because I thought that his death was caused partly by inadequate seating. I was told then that money was available for seating, but when the physiotherapist tried to get some of it she was told that I had 'misheard'. It seems incredible to people not familiar with physically handicapped people that chairs are so important.

My time at St Nicholas was now so taken up with the plasters and the Wombat that communication was almost at a standstill. Even Annie would sometimes go for a fortnight without a chance to use the alphabet board and, as the others saw me alone less and were slower at the board, their periods of enforced silence were made longer. By this time we had begged a talking-book machine from the Royal Victorian Institute for the Blind, and it was invaluable. The children could listen to books while I was bandaging on their plasters or giving them drinks or doing any one of the other chores that prevented my teaching them or reading to them. We began to get through books at a great rate. Annie read a lot on the page-turner, mainly non-fiction.

The Wombat was not entirely without its uses, and we were able to do some good work on those occasions when the circumstances were right. When Annie and Stephen were home in September, for instance, I stuck clothing cards on it so that they could both choose what they wanted to wear. They were able to use as many as eight divisions on the dial. Stephen worked the switch with his chin; Annie worked it with her foot. It was not the answer as far as free communication went, although Stephen was able to use it later that weekend to spell about half of his comment on a landscape exhibition at the National Gallery: 'Tasminnowm.' When I checked later on the alphabet board this turned out to be 'Tasmania v. English'. We still had to find a way around the problem that the children had in sustaining the immense effort of control required.

Nothing had improved at St Nicholas, and our relations with the Health Commission were as distant as ever. At the end of September I went to Sydney to attend a conference arranged by the Spastic Society of New South Wales on the system of non-vocal communication that they had developed called 'Signs and Symbols'. I found it immensely cheering. 'Signs and Symbols' is a system of symbolic communication designed for young children and intended to lead naturally to full spelling. It was not very relevant to the children with whom I was most concerned but, for the first time since I had started developing communication with Annie in April 1977, I was with professional people who understood everything I was saying and did not doubt that such things were possible.

I had been working in such isolation that everything I had been doing came as a surprise to the therapists at the conference. The Wombat and the circles were both simple ideas, and I could not claim any credit for thinking of them. Because I had not been part of the system, however, they were at least different from the standard methods in use, and I understand the circles system was taken up in New South Wales afterwards for use with retarded children.

After the conference I visited the speech therapy section of the Victorian Spastic Society, and I was shown a new way of organizing an alphabet board:

Diagram 19

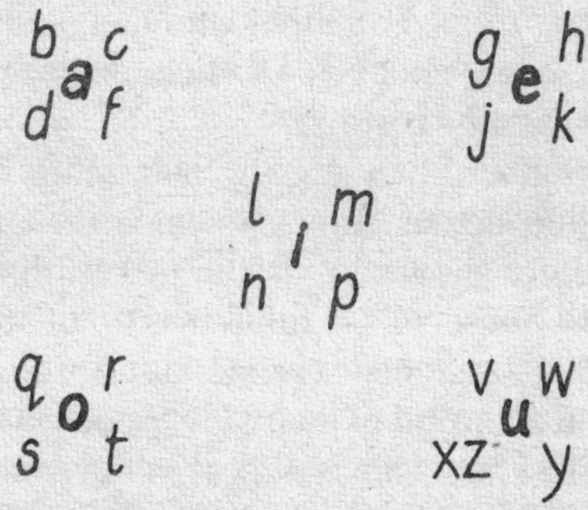

```
   b c              g h
  d a f            j e k

          l m
          n i p

   q r              v w
   s o t           xz u y
```

This arrangement meant it was possible for Annie and some of the other children to use a board unsupported. Using this board, the children indicated a group of letters and then answered yes/no questions to get specific letters. I did not persevere with this system and I should have. Annie could now spell a sentence in about ten minutes with her arm supported. Without support, we were back to the old days when a sentence took an hour.

A new wooden chair arrived for Annie in October, ordered at her request from some designers in New South Wales. It was not the most elegant piece of furniture, but it did force her into an upright position. It was also the first chair in the ward that came with an attached table, and it made communication much easier. I labelled one side of the table 'yes' and the other 'no' to help her in her dealings with other people. With the new board and the new chair Annie spelt out her first sentence that was independent of any arm support: 'Chair is going to be iklining [inclining] me to vanity.' All the nurses came to admire her; the chair certainly made her look older and taller.

Another recruit to the cause at this stage was Margaret Batt, a speech therapist with the Noah's Ark Toy library. She enthralled the children by telling them about a friend of hers called John Hickman who was a very badly physically handicapped athetoid who had managed to get his doctorate in mathematics. Dr Hickman was then working in Canberra doing research.

In mid-November I had to go to Sydney and I decided to take Annie and detour through Canberra. On Saturday afternoon we drove over to visit John Hickman. He lived in an ordinary house with a ramp instead of steps, and he drove an ordinary automatic car. He had an ordinary electric typewriter and an ordinary manually propelled wheelchair. And his physical handicap is almost in the same league as Annie's. His ability to live independently is extraordinary. The only analogy I could think of was Helen Keller living by herself without Annie Sullivan to help her.

Annie was shy with John at first, and she took a while to relax. He can talk, although he has obvious speech difficulties. Annie spelt, 'Tell us about yourself, please,' which drew him out a little, and she later interjected, 'Tension is a vast problem.' John explained that he had been given a lot of physiotherapy to teach him how to relax his muscles, and he gave us his prescription for rapid muscle relaxation when you are faced with a difficult physical task: a shot of straight malt Scotch whisky, a prescription Annie did not like.

His typewriter fascinated her. Annie asked if she could see him type, and he demonstrated his method. He held a stick in one hand to touch the keys while he stabilized the other hand by holding on to something. He was remarkably fast and very accurate. He was writing a book about the problems handicapped people confronted, and he let us read some of his manuscript which has since been published as *One Step At a Time*.

Our afternoon's visit seemed only to have skimmed the surface of what we wanted to say, and we were very pleased when John asked us to come back for dinner the next night. This time John picked us up in his car. His athetosis meant that the 'simple' parts of driving, putting the key in the ignition and fastening the safety-belt, were difficult for him, but when he got his hands on the wheel he could stabilize his movements and drive safely and well. Dinner was simple, cooking being one of the most difficult home operations. He ate with a fork, spearing pieces of food that had been cut up for him, and he drank through a straw. By the end of dinner Annie was visibly wilting. John commented that when he was really tired he got dreadful stomach cramps. That seemed to ring a bell with her. We tried to use the board with her a couple of times, but her arm kept going into cramp. Finally, just as we were leaving, I gave her a last chance, and with every ounce of determination she spelt, 'Thanks for showing me how to do it.' By the time she finished she was white. Part of her tiredness had come from staying awake the night before, when I had heard her crying quietly for a long time. The difference between John's upbringing and her own pointed out many lost opportunities.

We flew to Sydney and took Annie to the Mosman Spastic Centre. Annie used a 'Signs and Symbols' board to ask how much a wheelchair cost, and spelt out some messages on the alphabet board. I noticed that the staff members there were more lenient than I was about insisting on every letter. They could afford to be. They had confidence in themselves and their methods. One of the therapists showed us an improved form of the alphabet board with colour and position codes. Each letter in each group of five was given a different colour and five colours were lined up across the top of the board. To pick a letter you indicated a group and then pointed to a colour to show which letter in the group you wanted.

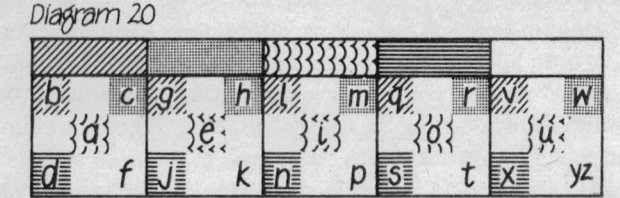

Diagram 20

b	c	g	h	l	m	q	r	v	w
	a		e		i		o		u
d	f	j	k	n	p	s	t	x	yz

One of the speech therapists managed to pick up a few words of Annie's, and nobody had any difficulty with her yes/no responses.

Annie joined in a group discussion with some of the children at Mosman: a real group discussion, with a therapist present for every child who needed help in communicating. It meant that all the children could actually talk together, rather than sequentially. The topic was 'What do you dislike most about the way people treat you?' and the answer Annie gave was 'baby talk'. The most valuable information Annie got from the day came when we were being driven home.

The therapists told us about the basic goals of physiotherapy: symmetry (holding your body so that one side matches the other), stability (having a secure sitting or standing base), and normalizing positions (using standard movements and postures). These were goals that Annie could work towards by herself and which did not need the participation of experts. I had never heard the aims stated so simply.

Chris took Annie back to Melbourne the next day while I stayed in Sydney for a few days. When I returned, I found that Annie had visibly improved physically since I had seen her last. Her progress was both amazing and depressing. If a few words and a few days could make so much difference, what could have been done if we had started years earlier?

Towards the end of the year DEAL began to blitz the politicians. We had lunches with local members of parliament and pursued anything that looked hopeful. One member of the DEAL committee thought something might be gained by approaching the new Director of the Health Commission's Mental Health Division, Dr George Lipton. We put together some material for him, emphasizing the importance of action if all this was to be kept out of the headlines.

On 14 December 1978, the day after Annie's mother had made her unexpected visit, Annie spelt, 'Vexing. Maginn [the Superintendent] didn't come yesterday. Tell him I want to talk to the Minister for Health.' I wrote a memorandum to the Superintendent asking for an interview for Annie with the Minister, and I despatched it through 'official channels'.

In the afternoon a big Christmas tree arrived, and I snaffled it for the children's verandah. We had a happy afternoon decorating the tree and listening to carols. It was very pleasant and the children enjoyed it. It was the calm before the storm.

The Director of Nursing arrived just before dinner, very angry about my memorandum. He said it was part of a put-up job, and that I just wanted to publicize my programme. He asked how Annie would know about the Minister, and he said that he was not going to pass the memorandum on to the Superintendent unless Annie told him what she wanted to talk to the Minister about. I suggested that he come and ask Annie himself. He refused but ordered me to take up the matter with her. After dinner Annie spelt out, 'Tell Bantos [the Director of Nursing] that I wrote to Maginn, not him. I want to see Houghton [then state Health Minister] without Bantos. TV does tell you who the Minister is.' I wrote another memorandum, this time to the Director of Nursing, in which I passed on Annie's message as ordered. Nothing more was heard of Annie's request. It was in a case like this that St Nicholas's equivocal legal status became such an obstacle. Because it was not under the Mental Health Act like most of the other mental institutions, its inhabitants lacked the simplest protection of the law. If St Nicholas had been under the Act the staff would have been obliged to pass the letter on unopened. As it was, they could please themselves.

On 20 December our political offensive reached its height. DEAL had a meeting with Liberal Senator Alan Missen and Labor Senator Jean Melzer, and a number of state politicians from both parties. At this point DEAL felt it had reached a stage where nothing further could be expected from the Health Commission, but as it was still trying to get help from various voluntary associations for the handicapped and government departments the committee decided to hold off going to the press.

We were also wary of publicity because we did not want the children's parents to find out about their children's intelligence from the front page of a morning newspaper. I doubt whether the Health Commission realized the hold it gained over us by not telling the parents. In any case, many parents learned about it in just the way we had feared.

We showed the politicians the State College videotape of Annie, and I spoke about the situation of the children in St Nicholas. It was decided that one state politician should approach Dr Lipton to ask for help and to see whether the committee could talk to the Minister. Everybody was worried about the parents and the politician promised to raise this question with Dr Lipton. It seemed very positive. But we did not realize just how powerful a bureaucrat could be compared to a member of parliament.

Our first feedback from the politician's meeting was quite positive: the MP had contacted both Dr Lipton and the Minister and had passed on some more background material. The next thing we heard came directly from the Superintendent: Dr Lipton had asked to see Annie's videotape. Everything seemed to be moving in the right direction.

I had produced yet another alphabet board, a combination of the Spastic Society's grouped alphabet, Mosman's colour-coded alphabet, and my original circles, and Annie was using it:

Diagram 21

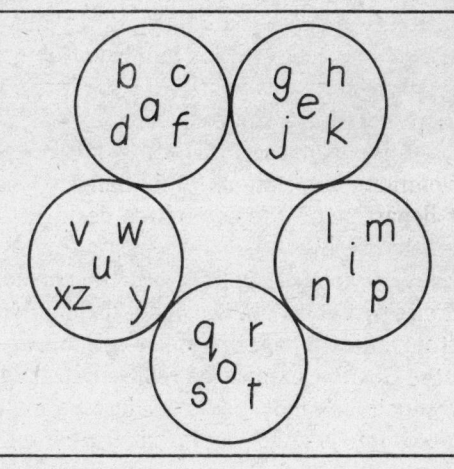

Each of the five circles was a different colour, and each letter inside a circle was a different colour from the others in that circle. To get 'a', for example, Annie pointed first to the circle containing 'a' and second to the red circle, because 'a' was written in red. Again, she had to point twice for each letter: once to indicate which circle it was in, and once to show which colour letter it was in that circle.

On 11 January 1979, Annie turned eighteen and spelt, 'I want to vote. Surely my IQ should not be relevant.' It is a fair observation. If we are living in a democracy, then retarded people should have as much say in their government as the intellectually normal. They could hardly do worse. On the other hand, anybody able to spell that out was not retarded. I collected a voter registration form the next day, and Annie made her mark on it after a considerable amount of practice.

Chapter Seventeen

Although things were moving slowly, 1979 had begun in a mood of low-key optimism.

On Monday 5 February 1979, everything changed. Annie had been tearful for a few days and unwilling to tell me what was wrong. On Monday she was tense and tearful for most of the day. She would not co-operate at meal times, and she refused to tell me why. During the evening meal she agreed to talk to me later about what was upsetting her. At six o'clock I took her out of her cot, and we went out on the ward verandah where the communications boards were. She spelt, 'Tell [Senator] Missen x put a pillow over my face on Friday night, but I screamed, and x got frightened.' Confronted by this horrible suggestion, I questioned her closely. Later I questioned the children Annie said had witnessed the attempt on her life.

I had no way of finding out the truth. It seemed futile to go to the police; I could not imagine how they could cope with the legal, medical and bureaucratic complexities of the situation.

On Friday I arranged for a speech therapist to visit the hospital. I wanted to give Annie the opportunity to repeat her allegations in front of an independent witness qualified in the communications area. The therapist was horrified and contacted the Health Commission.

Fortunately we had left for a weekend in the country with

Annie before the furore erupted. We did not hear about it until I telephoned Melbourne on Sunday afternoon. What we learned sent us racing back to the city. An inquiry had been set up, and I was to appear before it at St Nicholas next morning. When I told Annie, she spelt out a request for a lawyer. We did not realize the nature of what had been set in train, and we certainly had no knowledge of the way the medical bureaucracy would react when under threat.

The inquiry set up by the Health Commission refused to have anything at all to do with Annie. The inquiry members made it clear that they were not convinced that she had the ability to communicate and implied that I had manufactured the allegations maliciously for a purpose of my own. An action against me for defamation was mentioned.

The moment my two-hour interrogation had finished I left the hospital to consult a solicitor. I was refused permission to take Annie with me, but I was told that if the solicitor wanted to see her he could do so the next day at St Nicholas. I spent four hours that afternoon at Mallesons, a reputable city firm of solicitors, and I asked them to take on not only me as a client but also Annie. Whether they were defending me or defending Annie, they obviously had to see Annie.

Mr Graham Dethridge, a solicitor from the firm, came to St Nicholas on Tuesday morning. He had obtained permission from the Health Commission to see Annie at St Nicholas, but when he got there he found a number of obstacles. The Director of Nursing felt that he and several nurses should be present when Mr Dethridge saw Annie. This is not the usual procedure when a person sees a solicitor, and while Annie and I waited in another room Mr Dethridge rang members of the Health Commission to try to get permission to see Annie in private. Their response to this request was that he was at liberty to see Annie alone without me present, but if I were present, others should also be there. I felt that given Annie's means of communication it was a profoundly cynical response. Mr Dethridge finally got the Health Commission to agree that only one observer needed to be present, and that the observer could be someone on the staff who had not been involved in events so far. This seemed satisfactory for the time being.

The first sentence Annie spelt out was a request to see Mr Dethridge without the observer present. He felt that the only thing he could do was to leave the hospital and seek permission from a senior Health Commission official to see Anne without witnesses. I asked Annie if she had anything to say before he left. She spelt, 'Work to get us out.'

Annie's sentence proved later to be vital. This was the only occasion on which Mr Dethridge received instructions from her before the end of the action he brought on her behalf, and he had to rely on those words to support his contention that he was her solicitor and that she had instructed him. He did not see Annie again until three months later in a room in the Supreme Court building.

Annie's allegations had immediate repercussions at St Nicholas. I was forbidden to take any child out of the hospital, and I had to have a nurse with me whenever I was with the children. Annie had to have a nurse with her at all times. The nurses who were with us were instructed to write down everything that was said when an alphabet board was used, and everything I said to the children. In practice, it was less stringent than it sounded, because many of the staff could not read and write English well enough to follow the children's spelling. However, it increased the level of tension substantially and abolished the children's right to privacy. A number of children became quite distressed and were unwilling or unable to communicate under these circumstances. A further instruction was issued ordering me to turn over to the nursing administration the scrapbooks I had kept on the children's behalf containing cards they had received, craftwork they had made, photographs, and sentences they had spelt. I refused to hand over the children's private possessions without their consent, and I said that those who wanted the books should come and ask the children for them. This they were unwilling to do.

The level of tension around the hospital climbed steadily. Mr Dethridge persisted in his attempts to get permission to see Annie without a witness, but the Health Commission had contacted Annie's father who said that he would not permit her to be seen without a witness. Mr Dethridge appealed to Dr Lipton, Director of the Mental Health Division, and then to Mr Vasey Houghton, the state Minister for Health. It all took time, and Annie became progresssively more impatient. As I was no longer able to take children out, Annie and Stephen were unable to come home for any weekends, and Annie had to spend Easter marooned in the hospital. I was forbidden to visit.

I found it most unnerving trying to teach the children with two nurses watching me. As well, many of the nurses were not interested in what I was doing and would talk to each other or play with the children, distracting them from the lesson. Annie had to put up with much more from the surveillance she was under in the evenings and over the weekend. Extra staff were on duty to make sure she always had someone with her, and their interpretation of the requirement that they should stay with her all the time was that she should stay with them. Annie was put in her cot, her radio was turned on, but the cot was dragged into the playroom, where the radio had to compete with a television set going full blast and children screaming. Annie was constantly tired, because the night staff wheeled her cot around after them. When they were folding nappies in the bathroom, for example, she went along. I found her there one night when I returned to the hospital late to collect something I had forgotten. She was lying in a blaze of neon lights with three nurses talking and the radio blaring.

Several times when we came in with friends to visit Annie at weekends we found her white, scared, and tearful. She spelt out that she was afraid. She was not allowed to leave the ward at all until the end of February, not even to go into the hospital gardens. All the friends she had made over the past few years who had been coming to see her regularly now found that they had to apply in writing for permission to visit, and new visiting hours were devised to keep them away from her.

Mr Dethridge was still corresponding with the Health Minister at the end of March about going in to see Annie without Health Commission witnesses. He wrote:

Dr Lipton had referred to the fact that she is an informal patient at St Nicholas Hospital and has been placed there at the request of her parents.

We are instructed however that Anne McDonald was admitted to the Hospital at the request of her parents some years ago whilst a young child and has since attained the age of 18 years. Pursuant to the Age of Majority Act 1977 a person having attained that age attains full age and capacity unless he or she suffers from a deficiency of 'juristic competence or capacity that is attributable to insanity, or mental infirmity, or any other factor as distinct from age'.

As it appears that Anne McDonald's incapacity is certainly a physical one and that she has never been officially declared insane or mentally infirm we would submit that she has the capacity to instruct a solicitor and that we should be allowed to take instructions on a confidential basis in the normal manner.

Anne was becoming increasingly frantic. She spelt out that she wanted to see Mr Dethridge with or without witnesses. On 27 March 1979 she spelt, 'I want to leave St Nicholas. I can't take any more.' It was the first time she had ever spoken of leaving the hospital without the other children.

On 30 March the Minister replied to Mallesons:

Your letter refers to some matters of fact and some matters of law.

Ms McDonald's situation is well known to the Health Commission which is moving to resolve the problems in her best interests.

Miss Crossley, and other persons who are not employees of the Health Commission, have claimed that Anne McDonald has an average to high level of intelligence and the capacity to communicate through a technique devised by Miss Crossley. A body of senior and experienced professional opinion believes, however, that these claims are not well founded and that Anne McDonald is a profoundly retarded person (in addition to her physical disabilities). In view of the major difficulties in the professional resolution of this important matter, it is difficult to accept that Mr Dethridge is in a position to have any degree of certainty that Anne has the capacity to instruct a solicitor.

Because of the importance of properly resolving the question of Anne's level of intellectual functioning and capacity to communicate, Dr Lipton, Director of the Health Commission's Mental Health Division and an experienced child psychiatrist, has taken a personal interest in the matter. After reviewing all the available evidence he provided the Health Commission with a report in which he recommended, amongst other things, that an independent professional inquiry be established. The Commission accepted his report and recommendation and suitable persons for the inquiry are at present being approached. The Commission believes the matters relating to the various allegations referred to in your letter cannot be rationally considered until the findings of the inquiry are received.

I appreciate your reluctance to take steps that would undoubtedly involve Anne in unnecessary publicity and I hope that, in the circumstances, you will agree with Anne's parents and the Health Commission that a careful and dispassionate examination of the claims made about her will be in her best interests.

Because some 'senior and experienced professionals' said that Anne was profoundly retarded she was not entitled to have a solicitor to try and prove that she was not. The inquiry the Minister mentioned evaded just this point and ignored that the issues were not purely, or even mainly, medical, but involved instead the most basic civil rights and the most straight-forward concepts of common justice. A murderer awaiting trial has the right to see a solicitor without witnesses; Annie had not. No person can be condemned to a lifetime in gaol without having a chance to face his accusers in open court, to make them produce and defend their evidence in public, and to hear at the end judgment publicly pronounced.

Annie's parents had been told that she wanted a solicitor. Mr Dethridge suggested a conference, but they were unwilling to attend. It was becoming clear that permission to see Annie in private was not going to be forthcoming. Accepting this for the moment, Mr Dethridge arranged to see Annie in the presence of Health Commission representatives on 6 April. Just before the appointed time, however, Dr West, the Director of Mental Retardation Services, informed him that Mr and Mrs McDonald had refused permission for him to come and that accordingly no visit would be allowed. The Health Commission's way out of any difficult situation is to refer it to the parents. The parents, naturally, will usually ask the Health Commission what course of action it recommends and will usually go along with its suggestions. The McDonalds were not in a position to know much about their daughter or her ability to communicate. Indeed, I had been told the previous year that to tell the McDonalds about Anne's communication would be a violation of their privacy, of their right *not* to know what their child was doing.

During all this Chris and I had very mixed feelings. For Annie, the situation in St Nicholas was horrific, and her life there was totally miserable. She had decided she wanted to leave. Chris and I had not thought of bringing Annie home to live with us, although we had made it clear that she was welcome to come to us for holidays. We had been looking for an organization that would be prepared to take Annie if she had to leave St Nicholas, but we had been unsuccessful. Because of the political implications, nobody wanted to take her.

I fluctuated between rage and despair: rage that I was being dragged into worrying about somebody and caring for somebody against my will, and despair because I could not see any way out. Annie had made the allegations; I had passed them on in good faith. I could not now withdraw them in bad faith. I could not walk out with Annie, and I could not walk away without her.

It was horrible to see the effect that it was having on her. She was often pale, and she had black rings under her eyes as though she had not slept. She was always very tense, which meant that she had less control over her physical movements. In the six weeks or so that had passed since she made the allegations she had lost about a year's physical improvement. I was tense, also, and we kept having rows. I kept questioning Annie and saying that I did not believe her to try to get her to withdraw the allegations. During one of these confrontations she said, 'I bore people because the truth is so threatening. It is easier to believe I am lying. You are finding everything too much, so every new thing makes it easier for you to hate emotional involvement.' It was true. I was withdrawing.

During this period I felt as if I were dreaming. The allegations that Annie spelt out, the tactics of the Health Commission, the whole situation was something that you came across in books. It did not happen to people in the real world. It was like finding Dennis dead in the beanbag. It could not happen. On 4 April Annie spelt, 'I think that if Dethridge is ready to go to court that is the next step. Please tell Dethridge I feel sure he is competent to choose his clients.' April was something like a Rubicon. When Mr Dethridge was refused leave to see Annie altogether, with or without witnesses, we had to make a choice: did we go on or did we drop the case altogether? Chris and I decided that we were prepared to provide a home for Annie, and we chose to go on.

Because Annie had to instruct her solicitor through me, we made sure that there was evidence that I was not making up the instructions. Every visitor who did get in to see Annie asked her questions about what she wanted done and what she wanted to do. She either replied to the questions by using her yes/no responses, or if I was with her, by spelling. Their evidence was vital once we reached the court.

The situation was hardening considerably. I was no longer allowed to do voluntary work after five o'clock, when my official hours ended. I was also forbidden to visit St Nicholas at weekends. On Thursday 12 April I was told that Stephen would no longer be allowed to come to lessons and that I was no longer allowed to visit him at all. And I was not allowed to visit him to tell him that he could not come to lessons any more. Stephen's tongue had effectively been cut out. He would have no way of communicating at all. Stephen had not seen his parents for eleven years and there is no doubt that I was the adult closest to him.

Annie was very worried that she might be transferred to Sunbury, a large Mental Health Authority institution for retarded adults on the outskirts of Melbourne. When I saw her after Easter, all her belongings had gone from the ward, and the first thing she spelt was, 'I'm going to Sunbury. Fight for Stephen.' The hospital was swept with rumours that I was going to be moved out of Ward 2 and away from the children altogether. The rumours were not without foundation: my name was being shuttled hourly from ward to ward on the duty roster for days on end, and the Director of Nursing told me that he was only waiting for head office approval to separate me from the children and split them up into separate wards. When Mr Dethridge's permission to visit was revoked, he wrote to the Health Commission saying:

> As we believe that we have instructions from Ms McDonald that she wishes to leave the hospital permanently at the earliest opportunity, we request your advice as to whether the Commission will prevent her departure and, if so, the grounds upon which it would do so.

That was based upon my having passed on Annie's appeal to leave St Nicholas. Mr Dethridge was in the extraordinary position of having to trust me to relay correctly and truthfully the instructions of his client.

This was the first time that the Health Commission learned that Annie wanted to leave St Nicholas, and it must have sent some shivers through the establishment.

St Nicholas Hospital is in a difficult legal position. Children who go into St Nicholas are not certified in any way. No legal procedures are required. If parents ask the hospital to look after their child, and the hospital agrees, then the hospital simply acts as if it has the same powers as the parents.

A 1978 World Health Organization report on the law and mental health makes the point that children placed in institutions by their parents cannot be assumed to be voluntary patients, whatever their official status. It argues that children admitted by their parents should have the same protection under the law as any involuntary detainee: the right to an advocate, a permanent right of appeal, and regular reviews of their incarceration.

The Health Commission had never provided any such safeguards for the children in its care, and no thought had been given to the position of patients who had been admitted as children but had grown to adulthood.

The age of majority in Victoria is eighteen, and Annie had turned eighteen in January. Legally, her parents' rights over her had terminated and so, correspondingly, had those of the hospital. If Annie had been able to walk out of the hospital nobody would have had any legal grounds for preventing her departure.

Annie could not walk out of St Nicholas, and St Nicholas had no intention of allowing anybody to walk out with Annie. The contention was that as she only had the intelligence of a two-year-old she was incapable of forming an intention to leave, and therefore they were not keeping her against her will. Annie had no right of appeal to anyone outside the Health Commission.

Mr Dethridge had approached a barrister who had asked for an independent assessment of Annie's intelligence. Health Commission approval had to be obtained for this. DEAL had made contact with some reporters on the *Age* newspaper and gave them background information on the children's progress, not yet for publication, in preparation for the inevitable. A friend of ours had spoken to the state Premier, warning him that the situation at St Nicholas was likely to become troublesome.

The Health Commission delayed its reply to the request for an assessment because it was asking the permission of Annie's parents. When I told Annie this she spelt, 'What right have my parents to say whether I'm assessed?' It seems a basic point. If parents can refuse to allow their children to be re-assessed, a babyhood assessment could amount to a life sentence.

Our minds were taken off assessment on 26 April when we heard that Senator Jean Melzer had been refused permission to visit Annie. She went to the *Age*, and a reporter rang Chris to ask if the newspaper could use the background material DEAL had given it. Chris said the reporter could quote it. When I showed Annie the report she spelt, 'I'm afraid Jean may have fouled up my case.'

'Why?', I asked.

'Bad for judge to hear about it in papers,' she replied.

I reassured her that she had not been mentioned. On the same day we heard that Annie's parents had agreed to let her be assessed, the Health Commission had given its consent, and the test was scheduled for the next day, Saturday.

Two reporters were brought around the hospital in the afternoon, and the hospital put on its usual whitewash job. Dinner was not served until 4 p.m. and the nurses were instructed not to start putting the children to bed until the reporters had gone. Special education programmes, which usually stop at 3.30 p.m., continued until their departure at 4.45 p.m. I made a point of walking back and forth in front of the reporters a few times commenting on how nice the new meal hours were and how I hoped bedtime would always be like this in future, and I talked to the reporters outside the hospital later. On Saturday, the *Age* ran a front-page story reporting allegations that twelve children had been wrongly kept in a hospital for the mentally retarded.

The next morning I went to the hospital early to give Annie relaxation exercises while she lay over a large inflated Bobath ball, and to dress her in her own clothes. Dr Rosemary West arrived with the psychologist, Mr Bernard Healey, who had come to assess Annie. Mr Healey had looked at part of the State College videotape to give him an idea what to expect and what techniques he could use.

'Does she know her numbers as well as her letters?', he asked.

We talked for a minute or two about methods of assessment. Mr Healey said he would start by using the Wechsler Adult Intelligence Scale, one of the most commonly used adult intelligence tests. The Wechsler is usually given as an oral test, with the psychologist asking questions and the respondent replying aloud. Annie was going to have to spell her replies or point to them on a number board. The Director seemed nonplussed. She told Mr Healey that Annie could only communicate with my help. He said that he did not see that as a problem.

We collected Annie and took her out on to the ward verandah and chatted for a bit to put her at her ease. A nurse was in attendance. I suggested to Mr Healey that Annie should be asked if she had anything to say before testing started. He agreed.

I asked her, 'Do you have anything to say to the Director?'
'No,' she replied.
'Have you got anything you want to say to Mr Healey?'
'Yes.'

Mr Healey was able to interpret her yes/no responses very well.

Annie spelt, 'Stop Mental Health killing us.' I called the message out letter by letter.

Because spelling out responses is so much slower than saying them, it was impossible for Annie to do a complete test. Mr Healey was only able to give her selected questions. The test has many different sections, and he picked questions from all the sections it was possible for her to tackle. One test consists of putting jigsaw puzzles together, and there was no way to adapt that test to her capabilities. There were many general knowledge questions.

'Where does rubber come from?'
'Trees.'
'Name the Prime Minister of Australia.'
'Fraser.'

For answers of that sort Mr Healey would concede Annie the answer if she got the first two letters correct to speed the process.

'Name of the last Prime Minister?'
'Whitlam.'
'What is the capital of Italy?'

'Rome.'

'What would you do if you found a stamped addressed envelope in the street near a pillar box?'

'Post it.'

For the mathematics questions Annie used the number board.

'A lounge-suite was sold for $400 second-hand. That was two-thirds of the new price. What was the new price?'

'$600.'

'What is the population of Australia in millions?'

'Thirteen.' It was an acceptable answer.

'If you can buy two articles for 31 cents, how much would twelve cost?'

'186 cents.'

'If I can buy six oranges for 36 cents, how much would one orange cost?'

'6 cents.'

'What direction would you travel to go from Adelaide to Brisbane?'

'North-east.'

'An orange and an apple are both what?'

'Fruit.'

'The ear and eye are both what?'

'Sensory organs?'

'What is the boiling point of water?'

'100 degrees Centigrade.'

Mr Healey seemed stunned, especially by her speed in mathematics. The test provides bonus points for speed in answering mathematics questions, and despite the handicap of having to point to the figures on the number board, Annie was getting bonus points. We stopped the test at 11.30 a.m. on the understanding that Mr Healey would come back on Monday to do some other tests. He said he had enough information for court purposes already, but he would like to finish the test for his own professional satisfaction.

I was also stunned. Annie's performance had been completely error-free.

When Mr Healey returned on Monday, Anne started by spelling, 'I'm only a figurehead. Test the others.' The Director was not present, and the observer this time was the Senior Psychologist, Patricia Minnes. She had not seen Annie before and did not know what her yes/no responses were. The test went exactly as before. At one stage Annie arranged a series of pictures in an incorrect sequence. When Mr Healey asked her if that was her final answer, however, she said 'No', and corrected it. It was another error-free performance.

On Monday the *Age* ran another front-page story, most of it quotations from the submission I had made to the Schools Commission in 1977. No other newspapers showed any signs of taking up the story.

Tuesday was calm.

Wednesday began with an interview for a television current affairs programme, and later in the morning the Superintendent brought around a reporter from the *Bulletin*, a national weekly magazine. Dr Maginn watched as Annie spelt, 'I understand the *Bulletin* is very right-wing.' I went off to our solicitors shortly afterwards, and the reporter went on to interview the Superintendent. His answers give some insight into official thinking. He said:

We would love to have another Helen Keller on our hands. Do you honestly think that if we had twelve children of normal intelligence here we would keep quiet about it? I'd get an MBE. The claims are grossly exaggerated. All the claims by Ms Crossley are dependent on one thing – on whether any of the children can spell out a word without her help . . . Look, there is no doubt that there is a degree of communication between Ms Crossley and the children – but it is the claims for a high degree of communication we query. None of the children in question, I am convinced, is beyond the mental age of two. I have never seen any of them spell

205

a word without her help. In fact, I don't believe they spell a word even with Ms Crossley's help. Moreover, I believe that some of the children in her group have less potential than a large number of other children. We don't want any of the children to be used as a political club. Parents, to say the least, are furious. Imagine what it's like for them. Everybody's trying so hard in here, including Rosie. I believe she's utterly sincere. There's no way I'd stop her. I wish what she says were true . . . she's done a magnificent job. I'm the one that's always defended her over the years. We knew how good she was with the children – that's why we gave her the playgroup in the first place. But we need proof of what she claims before we can act.

It turned into a frantic day with the lawyers preparing affidavits and finished with a last-minute dash to get to the Supreme Court before it closed.

Her barrister, Mr Peter Heerey, briefly outlined Annie's case, and Mr Justice Menhennit issued an order calling on the Health Commission to show why a writ of *habeas corpus* should not be issued directing the Health Commission to produce Anne McDonald in court. We had a foot in the door. Nothing would happen for a week, and then the Health Commission would have to produce Annie or defend its failure to do so. Annie was going to have a chance to have her case heard.

Habeas corpus is rarely invoked, and the medical profession was being challenged by an ancient and honourable legal process designed to protect people from unlawful restraint.

Chapter Eighteen

We always thought of Annie's action for *habeas corpus* as 'The Trial'. Annie was 'imprisoned' in an institution and she was 'on trial' for her freedom. In a sense I, too, was on trial. So much of Annie's case depended on my evidence and, although I was not liable to confinement if the case was lost, I had no doubt that the Health Commission would dismiss me. I would be separated from Annie and the other children. Annie was being tried for her life, this time in a court of law.

Court procedure is a game played by gentlemen in accordance with well-established and time-hallowed rules. It is well-mannered, and manners have a distancing and disguising effect. We were fighting over someone's life, but the battle was carried on with a curious lack of emotion. Annie's absence from the court-room undoubtedly abstracted the proceedings. We were talking about an entity named Anne Therese McDonald, but few of those talking and few of those present had any notion of the person behind the name. It was easy to forget her in the process.

On Wednesday 9 May 1979 a friend drove me to St Nicholas, where I saw Annie and left her a bag of clothes. I did not know if Annie would be asked to appear in court, or if the case would be over in a day and she would need her clothes to wear home.

I left Annie and went to meet her barrister, Mr Peter

Heerey, in his chambers opposite the Supreme Court for a last-minute conference. He was waiting for the Superintendent's affidavit, which would be the best indication of the case the Health Commission intended to put, and he asked me a number of questions that I had been asked before. It seems to be a trick of the trade of barristers to probe in the eleventh hour for legal loop-holes, short-comings or fresh insights.

That morning, Mr Heerey found some very useful information in the correspondence files I had brought with me. I had been fighting since the middle of 1977, and I had scrupulously kept on file every piece of paper that was relevant to the children in St Nicholas. As it happened my files were crucial to our case.

The hearing was held in what is known as the Practice Court which is next to the main Supreme Court building.

In the court-room Annie's friends filed into two rows near the back, and the lawyers gathered at the bar table. The clerk of the court commanded our attention as he boomed out: 'The Queen and the Health Commission of Victoria, George Lipton, and Dennis Maginn, *ex parte* Anne McDonald.' Annie's case was to be heard before Mr Justice Jenkinson, who had been relatively recently appointed to the Supreme Court.

Mr Heerey opened her case. It was straight-forward: Anne was intelligent, capable of giving sound and logical advice to her lawyers and had told them that she wanted to leave the hospital. He argued that there was no lawful basis on which the hospital could detain her, despite the Health Commission's claim that her parents did not want her moved. Mr Heerey gave a brief account of the way I had developed Anne's communication and reminded the court that we were not taking sides against Annie's parents. As a summary he said: 'The applicant's case is that she is of full age, that she wants to leave the hospital, and that she cannot lawfully be prevented from doing so.'

The opposition's case was more complex, and it began with a flurry of technical legal arguments designed to establish that the case could not be heard because Anne had not signed the necessary certificate. According to cases cited by counsel for the Health Commission, Mr Gillard, the person applying for the writ of *habeas corpus* had to sign it unless it could be shown that he or she was under duress not to do so. Although St Nicholas had not allowed Annie to see a lawyer that was not duress, because duress involved doing something to Annie against her will, and she had not been shown to have the intelligence to have any will.

Mr Heerey retorted by citing cases which argued a contrary view, but neither side could produce a case that placed the matter beyond doubt. It was clear that if Annie's case was heard it would set a precedent. Mr Justice Jenkinson said he would consider the arguments while he heard the rest of the case.

Mr Gillard conceded that the hospital could not detain Anne if she wanted to go but argued: 'Bearing in mind Miss McDonald's condition and the wishes of her parents, the Health Commission feels that it has a moral obligation to ensure that Miss McDonald does have sufficient intellectual capacity to make a decision to leave hospital and that she appreciates the effect of that decision on her. At this stage my clients are not satisfied that Miss McDonald does have sufficient intellectual capacity to make a decision which is in her best interests.' He then announced that if the judge wanted to see Anne she was being held in a room off the court. I missed the next bit because I shot out in search of Annie. I found her in an interview room with an assortment of hospital staff and communication equipment. At least she had been dressed in her own clothes.

She spelt out, 'I have been brought here against my will.' By now the court had adjourned for lunch, and Mr Graham Dethridge, Anne's solicitor, had a chance to see his client for the second time.

Mr Justice Jenkinson decided that he did not wish to see Anne, and she was taken back to St Nicholas.

After lunch the medical testimony was presented, and Dr Philip Graves was cross-examined. The main argument centred on a conflict between a claim in Dr Graves's affidavit and a claim in the affidavit of the Superintendent, Dr Maginn. Philip Graves had said that Annie was an athetoid. Dr Maginn had declared that she was a spastic bilateral hemiplegic with the additional handicap of athetosis.

The significance of the distinction was that bilateral hemiplegia is usually associated with retardation but athetosis is not. Philip Graves was presented with a list of the typical features of patients with bilateral hemiplegia and asked whether Anne suffered from them.

'Does she suffer from motor impairment?'

Yes, he agreed, Annie did suffer from motor impairment, growth retardation, cranial nerve involvement, strabismus, difficulty in swallowing, and problems with tongue movements, all of which were put forward by the barrister as symptoms of bilateral hemiplegia. However, Dr Graves said, all these features were common to both spastic bilateral hemiplegia and athetosis. The features that separated the two conditions were that athetoids did not suffer from significant contractures and that when they were asleep the position of their muscles was normal. In both these respects Annie presented as an athetoid.

Dr Graves put a convincing case, and I was glad we were doing well, although I felt it was a sham battle. The real issue had not been raised. The flaw in the Health Commission's case appeared with particular clarity in an exchange between Mr Gillard and Dr Graves on the significance of Anne's early epilepsy:

MR GILLARD: '... it is significant, I suggest, that she suffered in the first three years of her life convulsions of *grand mal* type, and that that must affect your conclusion when you go on to say that these people can function at normal intellectual levels?'

DR GRAVES: 'No I don't.'

'You don't think it does alter your conclusion at all?'

'No, no.'

'So it wouldn't matter whether she had *grand mal* convulsions or not in that first three-year period? It is of no significance so far as you are putting forward the authority, people suffering from athetoid cerebral palsy can function at normal intellectual levels, is that right?'

'Yes.'

'In other words you say it has got nothing to do with it?'

'I don't dismiss it out of hand, but I think that the intellectual assessment of these children depends on the evidence at the time of their capability of communicating and expressing their ability. And not – not on anything that may have happened in the past which is at best suggesting that they may have a problem. We know that she has got a severe handicap, but I don't think we can extrapolate from that to say anything very definitely adverse about her intellectual abilities.'

It was as simple as that. The way to see whether a person was retarded was not to look at their history but to test them and see if they were. All that the Health Commission could hope to establish if Anne was a bilateral hemiplegic was that she was a member of a class most of whose members were retarded: it would be no more than a statistical probability. Luckily, the law is not impressed by statistical probability. It decides the question on the facts of the case before it.

Next it was my turn. I was luckier than Philip because I had had a chance to hear him, and his cross-examination had given me some tips. I decided that when I went into the witness-box I would speak up, look at the judge and answer no question with a simple yes or no.

Mr Gillard asked me how I taught Annie to read and how she used the page-turner, subjects I was used to speaking about. He did not question me on abstruse technical points involving my professional reputation in the way he had questioned Philip. I was examined on what Annie and I had done. All I had to do was to tell the truth.

MR GILLARD: 'What age would you expect normal, intelligent children to be able to read a book like *Roots*?'

MS CROSSLEY: 'Well, a normal intelligent child would be able to read a book like *Roots* in their teens.'

'In their teens?'

'Yes.'

'You seem to be able to achieve that in the space of what, about nine months, with Anne?'

'Yes, I am afraid that is so.'

MR JUSTICE JENKINSON: 'If one assumes that she does it with normal intelligence, she has the enormous advantage of escaping current primary and secondary education.'

Mr Gillard was building up to something. He asked me how I had established that Annie had read *Roots*, and what kinds of questions I had asked her.

MR GILLARD: 'If we were to ask her today what she remembers about the book, *Roots*, would she be able to tell you anything?

'Oh yes, I think she has a very good memory.'

'Who the main person was?'

'I think she would be able to – I should point out that she had seen *Roots* as a TV serial.'

Mr Gillard made a wry face and shrugged his shoulders. 'I was about to ask you that.' He went on to ask me how I supported Anne's arm, and Jon Hamer, a solicitor in Mr Dethridge's office, was asked to step out and sit in the box as a model. Mr Gillard asked some more questions about Anne's communication and gave me the opportunity to say a lot of things I wanted to point out. Our last exchange went like this:

MR GILLARD: 'Miss Crossley, have you explained to Anne what you want to do for her and you want her to live at home full time, in effect?'

MS CROSSLEY: 'I didn't explain to her. She told me.'

'Told you what?'

'That she wanted to leave St Nicholas Hospital and would like to live with me.'

'And do you think she has an appreciation of what is involved in leaving the hospital and living with you?'

'Yes, I do. She has a very good appreciation of that.'

It could scarcely be called a taxing cross-examination. Mr Justice Jenkinson asked me, as he had asked Philip Graves and as he later asked the others, some questions about Anne's communication. He was particularly interested in the possibility of an independent person – someone not known to Anne – being able to communicate with her directly, either by supporting her arm or by using her yes/no responses. He was clearly seeking information, and there was nothing aggressive or threatening about any of his questions. Our barrister, Mr Heerey, asked a question that really tackled the most obvious difficulty.

MR HEEREY: 'Miss Crossley, when communicating with Miss McDonald by means of indication of letters on the board, did you turn your mind to the possibility that you might in some way have subconsciously, or unintentionally, affected her indication of the letters?'

MS CROSSLEY: 'Yes, I certainly did. That is a major worry with anybody who is trying to facilitate the movement of the physically handicapped person in this way.' I explained the measures I had taken to the rule this out.

Sue Jones, our neighbour, was the next in the witness-box, testifying that she had been present when Anne had spelt that she wanted to leave the hospital and come and live with us.

After her evidence the court adjourned until the next day,

and following the usual post mortems I set off back to the hospital to tell the children about the proceedings.

Thursday's *Age* had a front-page picture of Annie, who looked very small, being carried from the court building. Once again, on my way to court, I took a bundle of clothes to St Nicholas before going to Mr Heerey's chambers.

Dr Maginn, the Superintendent of St Nicholas, took the stand. The examination began by recapitulating the core of the evidence.

MR HEEREY: 'Doctor, would you agree that there seems to be no dispute that Anne McDonald suffers from the condition of athetosis?'

DR MAGINN: 'That's correct, yes.'

'There is some dispute as to whether she also suffers from the condition of bilateral hemiplegia?'

'There's no dispute as far as I'm concerned. I'm certain that she does.'

'You say you are certain that she does, but you accept that a different view has been expressed by Dr Graves?'

'From what I understand Dr Graves said, he commented that Anne McDonald could have a mixed condition of spasticity and athetosis.'

'If I could put this to you as being in substance, Dr Graves's evidence: "I believe she does not have the condition of bilateral hemiplegia but if she does it is of a relatively minor extent compared with the condition of athetosis"?'

'That may have been what he said, I can't recall that in detail.'

'If you are correct and she does, in fact, have this condition of bilateral hemiplegia, as I understand it you say that it therefore indicates that she is very likely to be mentally retarded?'

'Yes.'

'Assuming that you are correct and she has bilateral

hemiplegia, it is a question of statistical probability that she is mentally retarded?'

'Yes.'

'Not certainty?'

'Not certainty.'

'And with any individual one, where there is a question of whether the intellect is impaired, the critical test is simply to see how the brain performs, is that correct?'

'Yes, yes.'

'And the usually accepted method for that is psychological assessment of the individual concerned?'

'That depends on the degree of development that the person has. It is impossible to psychologically assess people who have no form of communication.'

'Well, that seems to be what it is down to, Doctor. I put to you the statement attributed to you in the latest edition of the *Bulletin* magazine. Perhaps you could tell us whether it is correctly reported. You were reported (this appears in inverted commas), as saying, "The claims are grossly exaggerated. All the claims by Ms Crossley are dependent on one thing – on whether any of the children can spell out a word without her help"?'

'Well, before the . . .'

'Firstly, were you correctly reported in that assertion?'

'Yes, but there is – what I meant by "grossly exaggerated" are the claims that came before that, that is that these children are capable of doing very complex mathematics, they are capable of understanding French and Yugoslav languages and Greek and history and they even – Anne McDonald has taken part in another group with lectures on human anatomy, that's what I meant by being grossly exaggerated.'

'It really does seem to boil down to a question of communication, doesn't it?'

'Yes.'

'If the communication that she had with Mr Healey was genuine and not influenced by anybody else you would accept that that indicates she is at least of average intelligence?'

'Yes, yes.'

'And it would follow that your own view would be incorrect, that she would not be mentally retarded?'

'No, my view is that with the evidence I have now available she is functioning in, as I said in the affidavit, she is functioning in a severely retarded range. That doesn't imply that she will always be. With new evidence I may change my mind.'

In his affidavit Dr Maginn had quoted a number of times from Anne's clinical records. Her local doctor had said in 1964 that she was a retarded spastic. In 1965 the hospital paediatrician had said she had severe mental retardation.

In the years following she had a couple of physical examinations, and none of the doctors appeared to have commented that she was suffering from bilateral hemiplegia. The medical officer who had reviewed her in 1975 said she was profoundly retarded, and in 1978 the hospital paediatrician, Dr Basil Glaun, reported her as having a mixed spastic/athetoid cerebral palsy and had assessed her developmentally as having a maximum potential of a twelve-months-old baby.

MR HEEREY: 'Now, you have expressed your opinion in your affidavit based on your own observation of her and the study of clinical records in relation to her?'

DR MAGINN: 'Yes.'

'And I take it that in the study of those clinical records there is nothing that is inconsistent with the view or the opinion that you have come to?'

'No, no, there's not.'

'And if there was any . . .? Perhaps I could correct that. There is a statement in the clinical records made by a Dr Graves which does contradict what you have said . . . Leaving aside Dr Graves's view, the clinical records you say contain nothing inconsistent with the view that you have expressed?'

'That's correct, yes.'

'Your view, I take it, is that she is severely retarded and that she cannot communicate through this letter-pointing system in the way Miss Crossley claims?'

'That's correct, except my view is she is functioning in a severely retarded range. I am not saying she is severely retarded, that implies a static condition.'

Clarifying this point in a discussion with Mr Justice Jenkinson, Dr Maginn said, 'We like to talk in terms of a functional diagnosis of retardation. That implies the condition may change, the degree of retardation may change with other factors, or other information may become available at a later time, rather than to say that somebody is severely retarded full stop.'

Dr Maginn pointed out that the hospital had given me a place to work with the children, had given me a Possum typewriter and a page-turner, and it had set up a number of investigations. He claimed that St Nicholas had done everything it could to establish whether communication was possible:

DR MAGINN: 'We arranged an investigation by a committee, formed by – composed of Dr Roger Wales, Basil Glaun and the chief head nurse of our – Director of Nursing, Mr Bantos. Dr Wales recorded then, amongst other things, that he wasn't convinced that Miss Crossley's method of communication was without a certain amount of – he was in doubt about the method of communication by the moving of the arm. He did say, however, after a considerable investigation, that he thought that the children – well, Anne and some other children, could match words with pictures. Earlier than that we asked Mrs Vant, Jean Vant, to carry out a proper investigation of this, of the allegations that Miss

Crossley was making. She made a very scratchy sort of comment to the extent she was convinced the children were functioning at a better level than was originally thought. Well, my position, all along, Your Honour, has been that I must, as I am sure you will understand, I must be objective or more objective than anybody else. I can't appear to be agreeing with things because that may well make them appear more real than they are.'

The judge asked Dr Maginn at length about Anne's yes and no responses, and whether they would be able to be used for a satisfactory test. He seemed to think that they could, that if Anne had intelligence, she would be able to show it.

Mr Heerey returned to the question of the clinical record.

MR HEEREY: 'I want to read something to you. If you would listen carefully to this: "Annie has been seen on several occasions. I have observed her working with a magnetic letter board, both as the person supporting her and as the person who was asking the questions. I am satisfied in both instances that she did indeed answer questions, and in each case, had read the material and questions. However, both for Annie and the people working with her, this is a very tiring and time-consuming process. Also, unless one knows her well, and even then, interpretation when one is unaware of the expected answer, can lead to misunderstandings and frustrations for all concerned." Now, assuming for the moment that that is by somebody other than Miss Crossley, that would be inconsistent, would it not, in your opinion, that she is retarded and unable to communicate with anybody other than Miss Crossley?'

DR MAGINN: 'That's true, the latter part is true, yes.'

'You see, I put it to you, Doctor, that what I have read comes from the report by a Mrs Jean Vant, who had interviews with a number of inmates at St Nicholas, including Anne McDonald, which was conducted on 22 September, 1977.'

'Well.'

'Is that correct?'

'I don't know, I presume that she did, that she never seemed to regard it as being important enough to tell me about it.'

'Well, you say you have never seen such a report or heard of such a report?'

'No, not such a report.'

'It does not sound like the very scratchy sort of comment that you spoke about?'

'No.'

I knew what was coming.

MR HEEREY: 'Mrs Vant was Senior Psychologist with the Mental Retardation Service, was she not?'

DR MAGINN: 'Yes.'

'By 1977, she went to the Institute of Special Education at Burwood State College?'

'Yes.'

'I suggest she interviewed these four children . . .'

MR JUSTICE JENKINSON: 'How does it come about that you suggest such a thing, Mr Heerey, unless you are making application for leave to adduce further evidence?'

MR HEEREY: 'Perhaps if I could put the report first to Dr Maginn?'

The report was handed to Dr Maginn.

MR HEEREY: 'Would you have a look at that, please? Do you recognize Mrs Vant's signature?'

DR MAGINN: 'Yes, yes.'

'That is her signature?'

'Yes.'

'Mrs Vant is a highly qualified psychologist?'

'Yes.'

'Was there a Dr Barlow, who was, in 1977, Director of Mental Deficiency services?'

'Yes.'

'Do you know him and know his signature?'

'Yes.' . . .

'Would you read what that letter says?'

MR JUSTICE JENKINSON: 'What is the purpose of this cross-examination, Mr Heerey?'

MR HEEREY: 'The purpose, Your Honour, is to establish that this is a copy of the report that I read made by Mrs Vant and was supplied to Dr Barlow, and that Dr Barlow has indicated in that letter, and made copies available, amongst other people, to Dr Maginn.'

'You want to get Dr Maginn to agree that he has seen a copy of the document signed by Mrs Vant?'

'Yes.'

'Mrs Vant. Well, for that purpose, why is it necessary that the witness should read aloud the letter?'

'Well . . .'

'He has read it and he sees what you think will help to change his mind, about his previous evidence. Now, ask him does he now remember that he has seen such a report.'

MR HEEREY: 'Yes, sir. Having read that letter, Dr Maginn, do you now say that you received a copy of that report?'

DR MAGINN: 'Yes.'

'You did receive a copy?'

'Yes, I did.'

'That went into the normal records of the hospital relating to . . .?'

'Yes.'

'Did you consult that report in the course of preparing your affidavit?'

'Yes, but I still regard that report as a scratchy report. That is a one-page report.'

'It was a scratchy report?'

'That report refers to four children.'

'Why did you not include that report, Dr Maginn, in your affidavit, along with the report of other experts which tend to support your view?'

'Because I don't believe Mrs Vant – I don't believe that her statement that she – she's got – I don't believe her any more than I would Miss Crossley.'

'Well, do you think it might have been a good idea to let the court make up its mind about its validity?'

Dr Maginn did not reply.

MR HEEREY: 'The position is, that that report is, in your opinion as expressed, still unshaken despite the report?'

DR MAGINN: 'Yes.'

Mr Heerey closed his cross-examination of Dr Maginn. There seemed little to be gained by proceeding.

The next witness was Dr George Lipton, the Director of the Mental Health Division, who had little to say other than that even if Anne did have 'high cognitive functioning' she might still have defects that made it difficult for her to make appropriate judgements.

DR LIPTON: 'It is my belief, Your Honour, we're not to be assured that there is no distortion of judgement because of a variety of factors and some of these factors can be immensely misunderstood, even in those of full cognition or cognitive capacity, and I couldn't consider when that could be, at least not until one had a most intensely or detailed study by a variety of professionals.'

Mr Healey was cross-examined on his affidavit, in which he had said that Anne had shown 'at least above average intelligence'. Mr Justice Jenkinson quizzed him about the possibility of mounting an objective test. Patricia Minnes's testimony about testing methods was the only other evidence from the box. The judge also had affidavits from John Hickman and Dot Chandler about their communication with Annie. These were not challenged by the Health Commission.

Mr Justice Jenkinson was in a difficult position. He was retracing the problems we had been faced with over the past few years. We were in the court because we had not been able to find an acceptable method of assessment; if an acceptable method could be found it would relieve him of the need to choose between contradictory medical evidence and of making a decision on an unprecedented legal point about the burden of proof in such a case.

He had obviously taken the trouble to read the literature in the area. He was frequently able to throw the lawyers and, indeed, the doctors by displaying unexpected expertise in medical matters. But he had had only a few days to explore the possibilities that had occupied us for years.

'If Anne McDonald was put on the floor?', he asked Philip Graves, 'would she be able to move closer to the door from the place she was put down?'

No, Philip did not think so.

'Could she make two different kinds of sounds?'

Perhaps.

He asked me how long I thought it would take for somebody Anne had not met before to be able to help her to use the letter board. I didn't have any idea. He asked if she could hit a button, and I replied that she could if she were in a relaxed situation. Then he asked if she could do an unequivocal yes/no with her tongue. I had to say that unequivocality was in the eye of the beholder; I thought she could. He asked Pat Minnes whether questions could be devised that would be answerable by yes/no responses and still provide proof of intelligence. She admitted, after some hedging, that they could. Dr Maginn was asked whether Anne's motor control could be tested by asking her to keep her eyes shut until she heard a bell. He thought it could. Mr Healey was asked about one-way screens. I was called back to the box again for further questioning about her yes/no signals. I said that her tongue or eyes would be the most reliable signals.

But isn't there a tendency for Anne's tongue to protrude involuntarily asked the judge. I replied that there was, but that there was a difference between the involuntary movement and the one she uses for a yes response. I asked if I could demonstrate the actual movements.

The moment that followed is one of the high points of my career. There cannot be many people who have been asked to stick their tongue out at a Supreme Court judge.

Annie's barrister and the Health Commission tried to devise a test that would bind both sides. After some discussions a proposal was put forward for a neutral doctor to act as umpire in a test of the kind where I would go out of the room and Annie would be shown a word. We knew the hazards of that kind of thing: Annie might not want to co-operate, or she might be too tense to be able to do it, or her responses might not be clear enough on the day. But you do have to take risks sometimes, and the risks we would be taking if we did not accept were that Mr Justice Jenkinson might not feel that there was enough evidence before him to decide on Anne's intelligence or might think that if we were not willing to do the test it meant that we felt unsure of ourselves. We had agreed and Mr Gillard had told the judge when we found that the 'impartial' doctor who had been picked was not available and that I was not only to leave the room when the message was given to Annie but also to be blindfolded while I was working with her. It was redundant and impossible. I would not be able to say to Annie 'point again' or ask her to accept or reject a letter I thought she had pointed to, quite apart from the psychological effects such an arrangement would have on her. I went to the front of the court with a note to say that the suggestion was impossible. I need not have worried. Without pausing, Mr Heerey stood up and said we had changed our minds. It was so complicated that we were pulling out of the arrangement and were passing the decision back to the judge. With no great enthusiasm the judge agreed we had the right to do that if we wanted to, and the case was closed. He reserved his decision.

I had to go to St Nicholas and tell Annie that there was no news and there would not be any for some time. Our lawyers were pessimistic: they thought that we had the facts and the law on our side, but that it was a case that set a number of precedents. They thought that we would lose the first case but win on appeal. It was difficult to present this outlook to Annie in a cheerful way.

Back at work on Friday I discovered that the cupboard with the children's private things had been broken into while I was in court and their diaries and scrapbooks taken.

On Sunday the Health Commission held an open day at St Nicholas. I drafted some volunteers to stand by the children throughout the day to stop people discussing them in front of them.

The Health Commission indulged in some window dressing: three new colour television sets appeared on the Friday, and a toy library full of toys with their price stickers still attached was on display. At least open day gave all the people who had been forbidden to visit the children a chance to come and see them. The parents of some of the children discovered for the first time that their children were in the group claimed to be intelligent. The Health Commission had not told them anything.

Mark's mother had gone in to visit him and found herself watching him spell. After eleven years of thinking that Mark was profoundly retarded it was a shock. The *Age* quoted her as saying:

I don't know what to believe. I saw him point to the letters to make the words, but it all seemed sort of flukey . . . when you see something like this one day out of the blue it's just so hard to know what to believe. You want him to do it, but then you become sceptical after all those years of seeing him as something else.

Lesley, who points unsupported, spelt out to her mother,

'Take me home.' It was her first communication with her mother. Annie had been taken home by her parents.

On Wednesday afternoon I had a call from our solicitors: the verdict was to be handed down next day.

We gathered in the court on Thursday morning. Mr Justice Jenkinson assembled his papers and began to read: 'Return of an *order nisi* for a writ of *habeas corpus*,' he began. He went on through Anne's medical history in a detailed and an unhurried fashion, adding to every mention of her methods of communication the words 'it is claimed'. He covered the law and dealt with the question of her communication. He came to the conclusion that *if* Annie was communicating then Mr Healey's assessment of her as of above normal intelligence was justified. Then he came to me.

MR JUSTICE JENKINSON: 'It was not suggested in evidence or by submission on behalf of the respondent that Miss Crossley had manipulated the applicant's movements to achieve the selection of letters with the conscious intention of deceiving an observer. I was invited rather to attribute the selection of the letters, which it was suggested that Miss Crossley and not the applicant had made, to the operation on Miss Crossley's mind of her strong emotional commitment to achieving communication with the applicant and a similar commitment to convincing the respondent and others that intelligent communication by the applicant is within the applicant's competence. Although there was no evidence on the subject, I think that I should take judicial notice that psychological mechanisms of that kind may lead a person in Miss Crossley's position into deluding herself and attempting to deceive others, without conscious recognition by that person of what she is doing.'

It was not very promising.

MR JUSTICE JENKINSON: 'On the other hand, there was nothing in Miss Crossley's demeanour in the witness box to excite suspicion that she has been subject to those mechanisms, nor any evidence of conduct by Miss Crossley that would excite such a suspicion, other than her claims...'

The delay was tying me into knots; the judge had now been talking for twenty minutes and I still could not guess which way the verdict would go.

MR JUSTICE JENKINSON: 'The only other testimony against acceptance of the evidence by Miss Crossley that it is the applicant and not she who communicates is that of Dr Maginn. He is particularly well qualified to express an opinion on that question.'

The judge discussed Dr Maginn's qualifications, his experience in the field, and his opinions on Annie.

MR JUSTICE JENKINSON: 'The evidence of Dr Maginn merits very substantial weight. But the persuasive influence of the evidence in favour of the conclusion that the applicant is making intelligent communications has prevailed with me against Dr Maginn's evidence.'

Tears poured down my face. I could not even smile.

MR JUSTICE JENKINSON: 'Miss Crossley presents as an educated, intelligent woman of thirty-three, against whose good character and mental health nothing is alleged. Her testimony is supported by the opinions of a consultant paediatrician and an experienced clinical psychologist that it is the applicant's mind which is expressed in the selection of letters; and her testimony is supported also in several respects by the evidence of two social workers and a mathematician. On a consideration of the whole of the evidence, and of the probabilities for and against the conclusion that the applicant is the person who selects the letters by which communication is made when the applicant's arm is supported by Miss Crossley, I am persuaded that it is the applicant who makes those communications. If that be so, the conclusion follows that the applicant has expressed her wish to leave the hospital, for it was not suggested – nor would the evidence justify a suspicion – that although the applicant had a capacity to think rationally and to communicate her wishes, those wishes had been misrepresented in evidence ... The findings I have stated also lead to the conclusion that the solicitor and counsel who purported to act on the applicant's instructions in this proceeding did, in fact, have her authority.'

He found that the Health Commission was wrong in suggesting that an applicant for *habeas corpus* had to swear out an application or be shown to have been prevented by coercion from doing so. He found that her solicitors had been properly instructed. It was not up to him to decide whether it would be in her best interests to leave, or even if she were capable of deciding what her best interests were. He had decided that she understood what was meant by leaving the hospital. There was no evidence that she would be in immediate danger of serious harm if she left the hospital with me, and therefore no justification for deferring her release. If the Health Commission had wanted to give her extra protection there were other steps it could have taken. It could have invoked the Public Trustee Act or the Mental Health Act, and it had not done so. In the circumstances, he found no occasion for deferment of an order for issue of a writ.

Annie had won.

At that moment Mr Gillard stood up and waved a piece of paper that had just been brought into the court-room. The Health Commission did want to put Anne under the control of the Public Trustee. Indeed, it had just done so. Two doctors had seen her, declared that she was physically infirm under the Public Trustee Act, and a person incapable of managing her own affairs. What the judge should do, Mr Gillard suggested, was hold off on the issue of a writ while the Public Trustee and Anne's parents decided whether to set up a committee to decide on her future. It was a last-ditch stand, and even the judge seemed peeved by what appeared to be an attempt to evade the court's verdict.

Mr Justice Jenkinson looked over the certificates and said he would adjourn the case until the end of the afternoon to let everybody think about it, but that as things stood he thought he would go ahead and make the order anyway.

There is a long flight of steps from the Supreme Court buildings down to the footpath, and at the bottom there was a milling horde of reporters and television cameras. Walking down those steps was one of the hardest things I had ever done. I cannot remember any of the questions or my answers. The judgment had not been finalized, and the matter was still before the court. I could not comment.

Again I went to St Nicholas, this time with good news. Some of the hospital staff had been at the court and had got back before me. Everyone had heard what had happened at the court, but no one knew what to make of it. I was allowed to talk to Annie without nurses present for the first time in three months, and I took advantage of the confusion to see Stephen and tell him what was happening.

After a champagne lunch with Chris and friends, I rang Mallesons, our solicitors, to find if there were any last-minute changes of plan. They had been bombarded by reporters and gave me a list of people who wanted me to contact them.

In the afternoon I had to fight my way through to the court. Inside a barrister appeared for Annie's parents and made an application for an adjournment to enable them to form a committee for her protection, care and management. Mr Heerey opposed it on the grounds that the hearing had found that she was 'of sufficient capacity to make decisions about her own life' and that the order for *habeas corpus* should go. Mr Justice Jenkinson asked the McDonalds' barrister if there was any evidence that Anne's departure with me from St Nicholas would involve her in danger or immediate harm. The reply was that his instructions were that 'Miss McDonald's state of health is extremely vulnerable', but he made no other comment.

At this point Mr Justice Jenkinson said: 'I propose to make an order.' There was some discussion about the form of the order and finally the judge announced: 'It is ordered that the respondents not hinder the departure of the applicant from the premises known as St Nicholas Hospital, Carlton, in the company of Rosemary Crossley.'

When I went down the steps this time I had no excuse for not talking to the reporters, and by the time I got to St Nicholas reporters and cameramen were waiting there on one side of the hospital driveway. The Health Commission officials and doctors were on the other side. I walked between them, not quite sure whom I feared most. When I got to the ward I discovered that Annie had been dressed in the clothes I had left for her. Not surprisingly, she was very tense. She had been told very little. I took her down to say goodnight to the other children. I was worried about them, and I wanted to reassure them that I would be back. There were cameras everywhere, and photographers were shouting at Annie to look their way. One reporter distinguished himself by asking, 'Does she understand what's going on?'

I asked Annie if she had anything to say to the press. She gave an enthusiastic 'Yes.'

We moved out on the verandah, and she spelt, 'Thank you. Free the still imprisoned.'

I had to sign a form saying that I was taking Annie from the hospital without the Superintendent's permission, and then we walked out the gate.

ANNIE: I did not really believe I was going when the nurses changed me into my own clothes. No one spoke directly to me and told me what was happening, but I heard them saying Rosie had won. Quite a lot of the nurses did not believe it. 'Hip hip hooray,' one said, 'now we shan't have to feed her.' No one said they were glad I had won. I waited for what seemed like hours not sure whether it was true. By the time Rosie came I was too tense to smile.

No one said goodbye.

Chapter Nineteen

We returned to Errol Street to flowers and telegrams and a barrage of publicity, and Annie had her first television interview. Annie was asked whether there was anything outside the hospital that scared her.

'Yes,' she responded, 'people.'

'What did people do?', asked the interviewer.

'Stare,' replied Annie. And, once again, she told the world not to forget the other children in St Nicholas.

Annie's parents were hostile about the decision and a lot of publicity centred on their hurt and bewilderment.

Annie's release changed our lives almost as much as it did hers. Because it was so important that I stayed on at the hospital to work with the other children, Chris stayed at home to look after Annie for the first month while we looked for a suitable companion for her. It was a difficult time. Annie missed the rest of the group, and at the same time resented having to share me with them. Whenever I was at home Annie was happy and well behaved; when I was away she sulked, and Chris suffered.

It was obvious that anyone looking after Annie had to be prepared to provide more than just physical care. At the end of the month we were lucky enough to find the person we had been looking for. Donna Anderson had once worked as a nurse at St Nicholas; Annie and I knew and liked her. We decided to employ her to work with Annie during the day. Donna took Annie swimming once or twice a week, to concerts and films, went shopping with her, visited friends, and carried out the exercise programmes suggested by Annie's physiotherapist and the educational programmes I devised for her. Annie's page-turner and her television set came home with her, and she continued to watch the schools programmes and read the books she chose from the local library.

Annie's expectations of home life were based on her experiences of weekend outings and special occasions, and the everyday reality naturally fell short. This may have disappointed her, but she never complained. Her adaptation to our home routine was smooth. There was one exception to this: food. Annie did not know how to stop eating. She had never had access to more food than she could eat at a sitting. When she had come home for weekends she had been able to eat to bursting point at every meal with no ill effects; that was all right for one or two days, but she could not keep it up for long. If there was food in front of her she felt she had to try to eat it, and if you took away her plate before it was empty she would burst into tears even though she was physically unable to eat another mouthful without being sick. The problem has been recorded in survivors of concentration camps.

Not surprisingly, Annie began to grow. She grew up as well as out, and to her delight she had to get a complete new wardrobe. She grew out of all her shoes. A tooth fell out, and a visit to the Dental Hospital revealed that she still had most of her milk teeth. Her second teeth were waiting underneath to come through, and her dental age, we were told, was about nine. When another tooth fell out her second teeth began to erupt and come through in the gaps. Annie's body was like a clock which had stopped many years before but which started again when it was wound. Other cases have been recorded where children have grown dramatically when they were removed from deprived environments and fed properly, but it is almost unheard of at Annie's age.

Annie came home, but I had to stay at St Nicholas to teach. The rest of the children in my group were not given a moment to relax. Next on their agenda was the investigation set up by 'The Committee Of Inquiry To Investigate Claims About Children At St Nicholas Hospital'. The Committee, which had been established by the previous Minister for Health, consisted of four people: Dr Peter Eisen, a child psychiatrist, Dr Ian Hopkins, a neurologist, Doug McCully, a psychologist, and Gwenda Wilkinson, a teacher. It did not include any therapists, and of its members only Mrs Wilkinson had any regular contact with physically handicapped people or was experienced in the use of communication boards.

On 25 May 1979, just before the Committee of Inquiry met for the first time, Dr Maginn issued an edict that the children in my group should be separated to allow staff in other wards to evaluate my methods. Each of the eighty hospital staff members was to have a minimum of half a dozen sessions with each of my children. The children were moved at the weekend before I was told about the new programme. They were not consulted, and they were not told where they were going or why.

The official attitude to the children showed itself again in the method I was told to use in instructing the other staff: the Training Within Industry (Job Instruction) method, which was designed for foremen teaching process workers on assembly lines. I was to have one nurse as a student for each session, one child, and two nurses in attendance to take notes. During the two weeks this programme lasted the children had no education and no opportunity to communicate except when they were the 'subject' of a training session. I was also forbidden to visit the children out of working hours.

After two weeks the programme was abandoned because of staff opposition, not because anybody was worried about its effect on the children. I was told that I had a week to teach the children's yes/no responses to one of the staff (but not their use of the alphabet board), and that the children were to be left scattered over three wards. I was to be rostered as a ward assistant on the fourth.

I went back to the press. The Melbourne *Sun* went to the Health Commission and asked for its side of the story, and it produced three contradictory explanations. A Health Commission spokesman said I had coached other staff in my methods, and there was no need for me to go on working with the children. I had been transferred back to the job for which I was technically qualified, and the children had been split into different wards because the Committee of Inquiry had asked for the children to be separated so that they could be 'seen reacting to different stimulants'. This was just not true. The Committee of Inquiry had met for the first time only some days *after* the children had been moved. Under the circumstances Dr Eisen, the Chairman of the Committee, was forced to correct the report. The Committee asked for the children to be put back together in one ward. This was done (except, as before, for Stephen) but I was still not allowed to teach them or see them in working hours. Instead they were involved for about five hours a week in a baby development programme run by one of the nursing sisters. For this they were each paired with a child from outside the group who was profoundly retarded. Communication boards were banned.

It was in this strained atmosphere that the Committee of Inquiry started its investigations. Because of the changes in the children's lives, the members of the Committee never saw me teaching them, and when they wanted me to demonstrate a child's communication skills, they frequently had to retrieve me from the toilets I was cleaning in Ward 1.

During these months the children's only chance to communicate came when they were brought before the Committee. Members of the Committee did not seem to understand this, and they used to get annoyed when, for example, Stephen spelt out 'How's Annie?' instead of passing me a message. (At this stage Annie was not allowed to visit, and Stephen had not seen her for months.)

Even so, I was very happy with the way the children performed. Many of them were seen communicating by the Committee only once or twice for brief periods, some by only two members of the Committee, and most were never given the chance to spell a complete sentence. Nonetheless some excellent reading comprehension and mathematical work was done, especially by the older children who did not need their arms supported.

As the Committee's visits tailed off after two months I was restored to working with the group, at first for three hours a day and gradually for longer periods.

The Committee had written its own terms of reference and had done it so that Annie was excluded from its deliberations. They did, however, invite her to meet them. She saw them on 31 August 1979 and discussed the children's reluctance to work with them, suggesting that it was from fear of attacks such as the one she claimed to have suffered.

A letter to Annie from the publisher at Penguin Books in Melbourne brought on the next drama. He wrote to say that if, as had been reported, she was going to write a book, Penguin would be interested in publishing it.

Annie was eager to sign a contract with Penguin, but as her affairs had been placed in the hands of the Public Trustee he had to give his approval. This he refused to do on the grounds that Annie could not understand the nature and implications of what was proposed, and he failed to see, in his words, 'how he could be satisfied that the protected person could communicate to him' that she understood the contract.

As Annie said, it sounded like double jeopardy: her mental capacity had been attested to in the Supreme Court, and despite her having been put in the care of the Public Trustee only because of her physical infirmity, it was her mental capacity that the Trustee seemed to be questioning. The contract could have been rewritten to list me as sole author, and I could have given Annie her share of the royalties by some unilateral agreement, but I felt strongly that the book was as much hers as mine, and I did not feel able to write it without Annie being recognized as co-author.

The continuing correspondence between Annie's lawyers and the Public Trustee about the contract made it clear that any handicapped person whose affairs were administered by the Public Trustee on the grounds of physical infirmity was also envisaged as being mentally 'infirm' and ignorant of all worldly matters. Such a person loses the right to vote in Victorian state elections, for example.

The Public Trustee decided to seek the advice of the Supreme Court about the contract, as he was entitled to do under the Public Trustee Act. Similar problems were obviously going to arise every time Annie wanted to do something not contemplated by the framers of the Public Trustee Act. The Act had been designed for the senile aged, the retarded, and the psychologically ill who were living restricted lives; physically handicapped people were included more or less incidentally, but the same restrictions that were thought appropriate for other handicapped people were applied to them.

Annie asked her solicitor to request the Public Trustee to stop administering her affairs and to declare her not infirm. Mallesons provided the Public Trustee with a certificate signed by Dr Philip Graves stating that in his opinion Annie was no longer incapable of managing her own affairs and should be 'disinfirmed' (to use the dreadful colloquialism of the solicitor for the Public Trustee). The Public Trustee considered that he needed the advice of the Supreme Court on this question as well. The two matters were combined by consent. Both were thus applications by the Public Trustee for guidance – a decision in fact – on Annie's capabilities. Annie was not a party and therefore her lawyers were not directly involved. However, on request, Annie's lawyers were permitted by Mr Justice Murphy to be heard on the question of her capabilities.

Annie paid to put her case. The Public Trustee's request for advice would normally come out of her estate. So Annie was paying for two sets of lawyers to argue her case on opposite sides. There was little doubt that in effect the applications by the Public Trustee became a contest – The Public Trustee *v.* Annie.

Mr Justice Murphy saw, quite rightly, that assessing issues of fact was going to take up a lot of court time and would be highly stressful for Annie. Because there was provision in the Public Trustee Act for a Master to conduct an investigation, he referred the case to the Senior Master for a report. Masters are senior court officials (former barristers) who conduct lengthy and specialized inquiries. The application for the court to advise the Public Trustee on the question of 'disinfirming' Annie became an investigation by the Master of whether she was incapable of managing her own affairs, and hence an 'infirm person' within the meaning of the Public Trustee Act. The Public Trustee was, of course, represented before Master Jacobs but, instead of being neutral on the subject, the Public Trustee performed a role of devil's advocate, putting the onus of proof on Annie to show her abilities.

For this case Annie was given another psychological assessment by another psychologist. As the purpose of the test was to check whether Annie could communicate independently, the psychologist used what is called the 'Peabody Picture Vocabulary Test'. In this test, the subject must indicate which of four pictures best illustrates the meaning of a word said by an examiner. The words range from easy ones like 'cot' to hard ones like 'cornucopia'. We divided the top of a card table into four sections with white tape and numbered the sections from one to four. Annie indicated her choice by slowly moving her right hand into the area with the same number as the picture she had chosen. She was able to do this without anybody supporting her arm, something which she could not have done four months before.

The psychologist reported that even on a partial test Annie had achieved a score in the average range, answering sixty-eight questions correctly out of seventy-five attempted.

The first day's hearing with Master Jacobs was on Monday 10 September 1979. We left for the Supreme Court late and in a hurry. When we met Master Jacobs in his chambers, he suggested, considerately, that Annie might be under less stress in her home. He asked her if she would feel happier if he convened the hearing at Errol Street. She said she would, and he announced that we would meet there after lunch. A few more witnesses were heard before the luncheon adjournment.

Back at home the press sat on the stairs, television cameras filmed everybody going in and out of the back gate, Master Jacobs sat in the grandfather chair, and our undistinguished sitting-room became, for a time, the Supreme Court of Victoria.

Master Jacobs wanted to check that Annie had been able to answer questions in the way described in the psychologist's report, and he asked her to repeat some of the Peabody test questions, which, without her arm supported, she did clearly on the card table. The Master also asked some questions which Annie answered by indicating yes or no with her eyes, and he asked her to spell the answers to some questions:

'What is a contract?', he asked.

'Saying you'll do something and accepting certain conditions', Annie replied.

'What are royalties?', he asked.

'Funds distributed on a percentage basis for dramatic and reproduction rights', she replied.

It was clear that Annie was communicating, and I do not think that either Master Jacobs or the Public Trustee's lawyers doubted it. The next difficulty we faced was Annie's unwillingness to do the test that would have established it unquestionably.

The Public Trustee case brought to a head Annie's refusal to carry out tests that involved admitting the possibility that I was manipulating her, and that she was not an autonomous being.

On Monday afternoon, Master Jacobs sent me out of the room and said to Annie, 'What is libel?' It was something she should know if she was writing her autobiography, and it was a perfectly fair question. When I was called back in, she spelt out, 'I don't like any suggestions that my communications aren't mine.' It made her point, but it did not resolve the problem the court faced.

At the Supreme Court on Tuesday, I was sent out of the room and Annie was asked a different question. When I came back in she spelt, 'I think Ms Crossley is the least self-interested person I know.'

That evening she elaborated her objections to the test: 'Stubbornness is both my salvation and my besetting sin.'

'Salvation?', I asked.

'If surviving depended on any characteristic it was stubbornness: not letting the bastards grind you down,' she replied.

I believed it but I was not sympathetic. Whatever being capable of managing your own affairs meant, it surely meant being prepared to make some accommodation with the world and not destroying yourself on a point of honour.

It was fortunate that the Master's time was not occupied solely by Annie's refusal to pass messages. A number of witnesses gave evidence of Annie's ability to communicate and to manage her own affairs. Belief in one did not necessarily mean belief in the other. After Jean Vant had given evidence of Annie's ability to communicate, she said frankly: 'Whilst I am perfectly certain that Anne will become mentally and physically capable of managing her own affairs, I am not sure whether that time has arrived yet.' After Annie's stubbornness of the past two days I was inclined to agree with her.

Two doctors had certified Annie as an infirm person. One, Dr John Court, had written a certificate saying that by his personal observation there was 'no means of recognizable communication with her'; he was out of the country at the time of the hearing and could not be questioned.

Dr Bernard Neal, the other certifying doctor, had confined himself to noting her physical defects: her inability to sit, stand, walk, or carry out any 'purposeful movement'. He was questioned by Master Jacobs, who asked him why he felt that these physical defects made her 'an infirm person'. The Master spoke about Dr Neal's evidence in his report.

MASTER JACOBS: 'At one point in his evidence he opined that a person who could not move unaided from place to place, such as a paraplegic who could not get into his wheelchair without someone to help him, might be physically infirm under the Public Trustee Act. A moment or two later, he changed his mind about that, as it had occurred to him that a doctor might have had to declare the late President Roosevelt physically infirm . . .'

At lunch on Tuesday we adjourned until Wednesday

afternoon, when Dr Eisen, the Chairman of the Committee of Inquiry, gave evidence. The Master later described Dr Eisen's evidence as being 'of a general nature'. Dr Eisen appeared mainly concerned to delay any rapid decision. He suggested a number of other assessments – sight and hearing tests, for instance – which he felt should be made before Annie's ability to manage her own affairs could be determined.

I spent hours being questioned by the Master and the lawyers for both sides. I imagine the proceedings in countries that use the inquisitorial system of justice must be rather similar. We did not have two teams of competing lawyers with a judge umpiring; everyone seemed more interested in establishing the truth than in scoring points. That may have been because of Master Jacobs, who made it clear throughout that Annie's welfare was more important to him than legal formalities.

On Thursday Master Jacobs sent me out of the room and gave Annie a message. He had realized by this time that Annie felt that we were trespassing on her integrity, but Mr Justice Murphy had asked him to do the test. I came back, and Annie spelt, 'I know winning depends on answering the question. Solicitors don't know what life in an institution does', which was unrelated to what he had asked her to do. Master Jacobs asked us all to leave the room. Chris, Annie's lawyers, the Public Trustee's lawyers and I went out into the corridor, and Master Jacobs talked to Annie alone for a quarter of an hour. I think it meant something to her that he was prepared to do that. We came back in again, and I took her to the board. Even then she played around, consistently hitting the letter next to the correct one, according to the Master, still desperately holding on until the last. The Master asked everybody to leave the room except Annie and me. She spelt, finally, 'string' and 'quit'. I felt very foolish when everyone came back and I had to say what Annie had spelt. Everybody laughed unrestrainedly, partly from relief and partly from admiration for her bloody-mindedness. Master Jacobs had given her two words: 'string' and 'quince'.

The barristers summed up. The Public Trustee's lawyer refrained from discussing Annie's physical or mental ability to manage her own affairs and concentrated instead on her 'emotional immaturity'. As I am sure he realized, emotional immaturity is not one of the grounds under which a person may be designated 'infirm' under the Act. Annie's barrister gave a stirring speech based on an essay by Isaiah Berlin on Paternalism. It was all over except for the verdict.

I was worried. I did not doubt that the Master had accepted Annie as an intelligent woman, but the Public Trustee Act was so badly worded that I was not sure that this meant that she was not 'infirm'. When the Act had been drafted it had not been contemplated that the certifying doctors could ever make a mistake. I was expecting that Annie would lose.

A copy of the Master's report arrived from Annie's solicitors on Friday 21 September. It was not until I had been home for an hour that Chris said very glumly, 'There's something you'd better read.' My heart sank. I read very slowly through the details of the hearing, trying to postpone the inevitable disappointment. Here it was: 'My conclusion is that Miss McDonald is not infirm within the meaning of Section 39(c) of the Public Trustee Act.' Chris, who has a mordant sense of humour, was laughing at the expression on my face. Annie had won again.

Master Jacob's report showed all the concern for Annie's future that he had shown during the inquiry.

He talked not only of her intellectual and communication abilities but also of the obvious changes in her since she had left St Nicholas:

MASTER JACOBS: 'Since May 1979, Miss McDonald has

grown, physically, to the size of a seven to eight year old. Her weight has doubled in the past two years. She is now losing her "milk" teeth and getting her second teeth.'

His report was, if anything, too nice about me.

MASTER JACOBS: 'Miss Crossley's demeanour throughout, and her answers under cross-examination, and to me, completely satisfied me that she is an honest person, with a sincere desire to help, rather than to exploit her protégée. Not only did I form that opinion of her, but also the opinion that she has a genuine dedication towards the goal of improving the lives of cerebral palsy victims in general, as well as that of Anne McDonald in particular. Her talents and abilities in that direction are, I believe, very considerable. That is not to say that she is oblivious to the possibility that she may make a personal gain. She conceded that she may do so. But I am quite satisfied that if any such motive exists it is of a secondary nature, and that she has not set out to exploit Miss McDonald. The arrival at such a conclusion about Miss Crossley has an important bearing on the question of whether Miss McDonald is able, in the circumstances in which she is now placed, to manage her own affairs.'

The report dealt very sensitively with the problems of Annie's parents:

MASTER JACOBS: 'One can understand and sympathize with the feelings of parents who have for eighteen years lived in the sincere belief that their child is hopelessly mentally retarded, and how hard it must be for them to accept the fact that for many years they have parted with a person who possesses a real intellect. It is to be earnestly hoped that Miss McDonald's intellect will eventually become so apparent that her parents, too, will recognize it, and will then experience the joy of a new relationship with their daughter.'

Mr Justice Murphy still had to make his decision.

Although he would be guided by the Master's report, he was not obliged to follow its recommendations. Judgement day was Tuesday 25 September. While we were waiting, the Public Trustee told us that he would not be taking his costs out of Annie's estate. Legal Aid later agreed to pay Anne's costs.

Mr Justice Murphy detailed the circumstances of the case; he recapitulated Mr Justice Jenkinson's findings, and praised the Master's report. He discussed the report in some detail. He had obviously thought about it deeply.

MR JUSTICE MURPHY: 'This case has aroused public interest, for it is no doubt a case in which some of the accepted norms of our society may appear to be challenged; as a consequence of the inquiries which have been instituted, a reappraisal of the tests by which, in the past, it has often been adjudged that a human being is not capable of managing his or her own affairs may be called for. However, the issue is certainly a complex one. In the present case there is no suggestion of mental infirmity made at all. The physical infirmities are obvious to the world. The question then becomes – do those physical infirmities in the circumstances cause Miss McDonald to be incapable of managing her own affairs?'

He went on to say: 'Miss McDonald appears to me to be clearly to be unable to fend for herself in any normal way, but I accept that she is able to communicate with Miss Crossley and with a limited number of people, perhaps being those who are prepared to take the trouble and to spend the time necessary to achieve this end.'

This was his conclusion.

MR JUSTICE MURPHY: 'I will order the Public Trustee to sign and seal a certificate in the form of the Fifth Schedule to the Public Trustee Act 1958 that Miss Anne Therese McDonald has ceased to be an infirm person for the purposes of the Public Trustee Act 1958.'

After two Supreme Court hearings, Annie had won full human rights.

ANNIE: Moving out of St Nicholas and into an ordinary home made me aware for the first time how little I know about the real world. When we came at weekends it was an outing. Chris and Rose had prepared everything in advance, and we didn't see the work which went into making sure we had a good time. For uninitiated visitors it seemed there was no work involved in running a house. Our dishes and clothes were washed after we left. The house was cleaned before we came.

Seeing Rosie wash my clothes every night made me realize what she was sacrificing for me. As well there was the cost; all of Rosie's salary was used to pay Donna, which meant the household income was halved.

After I left St Nicholas I wasn't allowed to visit the others for some time. This really distressed me. I felt I had deserted them. When I saw them in the garden across the road from the hospital I burst into tears. It seemed so unfair that only one of us was getting a chance. Why wasn't the Health Commission prepared to give them the benefit of the doubt? The saddest thing since leaving has been not being able to help the others.

Social life was one thing I missed. At St Nicholas I had my friends with me all the time. It took me some time to get used to the ordinary system where you see your friends at intervals varying from days to months. I gradually made friends, more so than when I had come for weekends. What really pleased me was when I started being asked out without Chris and Rosie. I felt I was no longer an appendage but a person in my own right. Dining with Chris and Rosie at a French restaurant with Dr Lipton at the next table showed me how much my circumstances had changed.

It was difficult to avoid clinging to Rosie. Suddenly being

raced from babyhood to adulthood does have its drawbacks. I was being given a chance, but I had enormous worries. Would I be accepted in the outside world? Everybody was saying that Rosie wouldn't be able to cope and I'd be back in St Nicholas in a month. How would Chris like me living with them? Did they realize how much work I was? I needed to be reassured constantly that they loved me and would keep me regardless of how I behaved. This often resulted in my behaving atrociously in order to test them.

With the first year gone my doubts seem absurd. Chris and Rosie wistfully complain that they get less at birthdays than they used to, but I get given more, so it all evens out. Three can live as happily as two.

Epilogue

On 30 April 1980 the Committee of Inquiry's report was tabled in Parliament. I saw it first when I came to the hospital after taking Phillip swimming. Reporters waylaid me in the garden. When they realized I hadn't read it, they suggested I sit down on one of the benches and passed me a copy open at the Committee's conclusions.

The Committee had found:

Not one of the 11 children shows any evidence of a level of intellectual functioning beyond that expected of children of two and a half to three years of age. The 11 children function at levels indicative of severe or profound mental retardation.

There is no valid evidence to support the claims that these children can communicate by the use of an alphabet board. Ms Crossley's claims that these children are capable of understanding and communicating highly sophisticated concepts are false. No child shows evidence of even the most elementary level of literacy or numeracy.

The Committee recommended:

As the 11 children function at levels indicative of severe and profound mental retardation Ms Crossley's educational program is inappropriate and should be immediately discontinued.

As the consequences of Ms Crossley's incorrect judgements and perceptions are likely to be harmful to these children, she should have no continuing formal contact with them.

Because of Ms Crossley's attitudes towards other staff and the parents of these children, it is inappropriate that she should continue to work at St Nicholas Hospital.

At first I could scarcely take it in. Although we had all thought that the Committee might be too timid to make a positive finding, the weight of the evidence was such that the worst we had envisaged was a fence-sitting report recommending further investigation. Suddenly the foundations on which my world was based had shifted.

Fortunately, the media had deadlines, and after I had made some incoherent comments they went away. I was left to tell the children and to say goodbye. I told them that the report's conclusions were as bad as could be, but that we would contest them. I did not realize how powerless we were.

The report was a mixture of smears, innuendoes, twisted logic, glaring omissions and outright lies, but it had been tabled in Parliament, and its authors were able to shelter behind the cloak of parliamentary privilege. Neither I nor any of the other people defamed in the document had any redress. The Supreme Court had twice corrected the mistakes of the medical profession. This time it was powerless. No legal action is possible against a document that has been tabled in Parliament, and there is no appeal. That document can be quoted against the children and me for the rest of ours lives, and we have no defence. The truth of the allegations is not relevant.

Only two of the group had been given formal psychological assessments – the others were presumably found guilty by association – and the two who were tested were not allowed to use their communication boards; the psychologists thought it was a 'time-consuming' and 'very restricted' method of communication.

The Committee did ask some of the children to pass messages, as the Master did with Anne; most of the children who were asked refused, and what success was achieved went unreported. Existing objective evidence, such as that from Roger Wales's tests, was ignored totally, as were those sessions where children communicated without having their arms supported.

The Committee received submissions from various professional bodies – the Australian Psychological Society, the Spastic Society, the State Association for the Retarded – but their views were disregarded. Wesley Central Mission offered places at one of its homes to three of the group so that a long-term education and evaluation programme could be provided for them. The Committee ignored the offer and informed the Minister that there was no alternative accommodation for any of the children outside the hospital.

Despite the repeated requests of all the professionals associated with the children, the Committee did not obtain the help of any therapists experienced with severe communication problems. It was pointed out repeatedly that to demand independent communication from children when they had been denied all the facilities necessary for independent communication – chairs, therapy, technology – was to put the cart before the horse.

The Committee condemned me, but it could not entirely acquit St Nicholas, however hard it tried:

The facilities of the hospital are less than optimal for the care of grossly (*sic*) handicapped children . . . There is a gross shortage of available and optimal seating and support furniture and equipment. It is evident that *the prevention of musculo-skeletal deformities* (my italics) and the facilitation of response to . . . educational programs would be enhanced if the children had individualized seating and support equipment . . .

The children wear somewhat uniform clothing, may be toileted in the presence of others, and go to bed in the late afternoon or early evening. Whether these are wrong, harmful, dangerous, degrading or insulting practices seems to depend on the attitudes, viewpoints, knowledge, experience or skills of the critics. The

Committee did not observe any evidence of adverse effects from these practices.

A most telling sentence in the Committee's report read, 'No child showed emotions of shame, doubt, or guilt ...' The Committee did not say why it thought the children should feel ashamed or guilty. Should they be ashamed because they were put to bed in the late afternoon, because they did not have clothes of their own, because they were not allowed to visit or be visited by their friends, because they were in nappies and were changed in public, because they had no wheelchairs, because they had no therapy, because they do not have the right to communicate, because they have preventable skeletal deformities? Whoever should be ashamed it is not these children. After burning their records at the suggestion of the Health Commission, the Committee members returned to their jobs in the Education Department or in Health Commission hospitals.

Professional feeling against the report was strong, and a public meeting convened at an advanced education college nominated two psychologists, Dr Robert Cummins and Ms Heather Bancroft, to investigate the conduct of the Committee.

After the Committee's report was released I was immediately transferred to the Health Commission library and banned from visiting St Nicholas. Angela Wallace attempted to initiate an action for *habeas corpus*, but this fell through when the church which had been going to provide her with accommodation declared in response to pressure and publicity that they would not accept any disabled person, regardless of age and intelligence, without his or her parents' permission. This Angela's parents were not prepared to give. The Health Commission approached the parents of the rest of the group and requested that they hand control of their children over to the hospital. Consent or failure to reply was taken as a licence to ban all visitors (apart from the parents, who by and large were not visiting anyway). Communication boards were banned.

Outside we did what we could. We lobbied. We fought battles in the media. We published the first edition of this book. Some things did change. At the end of 1980 a long-standing promise to separate Mental Retardation Services from Mental Health was implemented. Errol Cocks, a psychologist, came from interstate to be the first director of the new division. He had liberal views about disabled people and their rights and no stake in the current controversy. Although he was unable to bring any immediate changes in the situation at St Nicholas, he was able to get the government to accept a long-term solution.

By September 1981 the review of the Committee of Inquiry's findings had been completed by Dr Cummins and Ms Bancroft, and arrangements had been made for their report to be released by Victoria's shadow Health Minister, Tom Roper. It was critical not only of the Committee's methods but also of conditions at St Nicholas. Release day was Monday, 7 September 1981. On the preceding Friday the Health Minister announced that St Nicholas would be closed. The residents would all be housed in small groups in ordinary houses scattered throughout the community. The hospital would be razed and the site sold. The money provided by this sale, of what was, after all, prime inner city land, would pay for the rehousing.

With that announcement, and the release of the Burwood report, it appeared that the battle was all over. After we left Parliament House on Monday, I went to St Nicholas. I wasn't allowed past the enquiry desk, but I left some flowers for Stephen with a note, 'St Nicks is coming down and you'll be coming out.' Late that night Stephen died.

ANNE: Stephen's death was the end of my belief in God. Previously I had wanted to believe in a caring God, who could love even people like us. No one who loved Stephen could have let him die a prisoner of his own body and of the Health Commission.

Stephen had been allowed no visitors in the year before he died. He had no way of complaining, no way of communicating. He was not allowed to leave the hospital. His mail was interfered with. He was a political prisoner. It was heartbreaking to be forever unsure of what he knew. Did he think he had been abandoned? Did he know how much he was loved and how we were working to free him?

I am out, but I can never forget that others are waiting. Lesley Waddingham died in 1982 and Mark Corkhill died in 1983. St Nicholas has still not been closed. Everything I have done only emphasizes the difference between my opportunities and those of the survivors.

Since leaving I have grown 40 centimetres. Now I sit in an ordinary wheelchair and use a pointer mounted on a headband to operate a mini-typewriter or a voice-synthesizer. In 1981 I sat a public exam in English and passed. In 1983 I started a Humanities degree and completed two units. At the end of 1983 I was given a grant by the Australia Council to work on a book about the ethics of the decisions the community makes about its disabled members. I no longer receive a pension but am a taxpayer entitled to complain about my hard-earned money being used to support severely disabled children who will never contribute.

Some things have not changed. I still feel I should not have been resuscitated given that I was destined to be institutionalized. My parents do not visit. I think they refuse to see me type for fear that this book may all be true.

While being out has enabled me to grow in body I am not sure whether I have matured emotionally. I am still very possessive and hate sharing people. When meeting people for the first time I often become so shy I am unable to communicate. From the floor at St Nicholas to chatting with

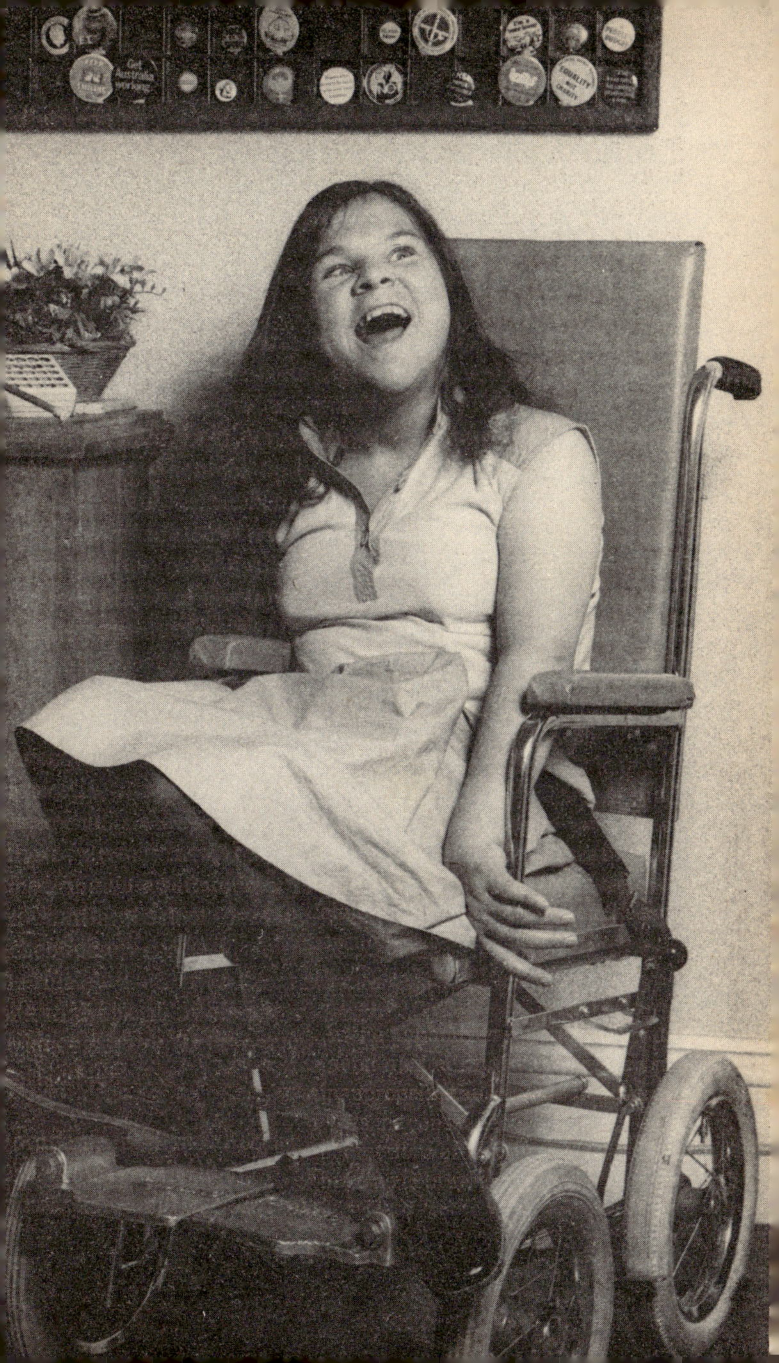
Get Australia working
EQUALITY NOT CHARITY

a Minister of State is a long jump, and I seem to have missed the ground in between. I have been expected to behave either like an animal or an ambassador when better casting would give me a part as an adolescent.

Puberty, like my growth, is delayed. This makes for difficulties in what would otherwise be sexual relationships. I may not be a Peta Pan for the rest of my life, but now I am an adult with a child's body. It is interesting to speculate on what changes puberty might bring to my cognitive processes.

Being a disabled person is not all bad. At twenty-three I have probably done more than I would have had I grown up as a normal girl in a country town. Soon a film based on this book is to be released, and although I had grown too much to play the part myself I was able to participate in its making. I have watched myself portrayed on stage in three plays also based on this book. I have met some remarkable people and made some wonderful friends. And no one ever asks me to do the washing-up.

Throughout these years I have lived with Chris and Rosie. We fight continuously, and each calls the other two stupid, ill mannered and obese. There is some justice in this as far as Chris and Rose are concerned. Generally, however, they aren't bad – I might even say they're magnificent.

ROSEMARY: Since Anne has left St Nicholas we have all become more aware of the wider community of people with disabilities and have worked with it to break down the barriers of ignorance and prejudice which exist not only between non-disabled and disabled people, but also between people with different disabilities. These days we no longer talk about 'beanbaggers' because that is a stigmatizing label. Anne will never again wear her badge saying 'I'm handicapped not stupid' because it denigrates her friends who are intellectually disadvantaged.

Since resigning from the Health Commission library in 1982 I have become especially concerned about the plight of people who sustain severe brain damage as the result of accidents. If they lose speech and movement, as many do, they are just as vulnerable to misdiagnosis as any baby with cerebral palsy. My work with people who have had head injuries has lead me to revise my approach to communication boards.

I looked for ways to enable people to point clearly with small movements. Even very limited head movement can enable a person to use a headpointer to type on a Canon Communicator, a sort of micro-typewriter that produces paper tape. Anne, Sharon, young Mark, and both Angelas can all use one. If I had not been so isolated from other people working on non-vocal communication I would have discovered this years ago.

At the end of 1982 a new Director of Nursing was appointed to St Nicholas, and since then the improvements that started slowly in 1980 have speeded up, and restrictions on visiting have been relaxed, although not repealed. Prolonged efforts by many people have led to the establishment of a special communication programme at Dame Mary Herring Spastic Centre for Leonie, Noelene, Phillip and Sharon, in which I participate as a teacher.

Angela Wallace is still trying to challenge the verdict of the Committee of Inquiry in the courts. Before starting an unsuccessful action she typed, 'I want to be allowed to communicate what, when, where, how, and to whom I wish.'

Free speech is an impossibility for Anne and people like her. Freedom of expression is not impossible, but it is exceedingly vulnerable, because it is always dependent on the co-operation of others. Voltaire said, 'I disapprove of what you say, but I will defend to the death your right to say it.' To wilfully deprive any person of that right is to endanger the liberty of us all. Democracy is the first victim of censorship, humanity the second. While the rights of people with disabilities are dependent on the arbitrary exercise of generosity by the rest of us, we are repudiating their humanity, their right to a life worth living.